Study Guide for

Pathophysiology:

A Clinical Approach

SECOND EDITION

Study Guide for

Pathophysiology:

A Clinical Approach

Carie Braun, PhD, RN

Cindy Anderson, PhD, RN, WHNP-BC, FAAN

Contributing Writer: Julie Strelow, MSN, RN

Wolters Kluwer | Lippincott Williams & Wilkins
Health

Philadelphia • Baltimore • New York • London
Buenos Aires • Hong Kong • Sydney • Tokyo

Acquisitions Editor: David B. Troy
Associate Product Manager: Erin M. Cosyn
Product Director: Tanya M. Martin
Marketing Manager: Allison Powell
Designer: Paul Fry
Compositor: MPS Limited, a Macmillan Company
Printer: Data Reproductions Corporation

To purchase additional copies of this book, call our customer service department at **(800) 638-3030** or fax orders to **(301) 223-2320**. International customers should call **(301) 223-2300**.

Visit Lippincott Williams & Wilkins on the Internet: http://www.LWW.com. Lippincott Williams & Wilkins customer service representatives are available from 8:30 am to 6:00 pm, EST.

11
2 3 4 5 6 7 8 9 10

This is the Study Guide to accompany Braun and Anderson's *Pathophysiology: A Clinical Approach*. It is a learning resource that will help you retain important information and comprehend basic functions and processes of the human body. To help you get the most out of your studies, this Study Guide offers a variety of exercises that will help reinforce the material you have learned and build your critical-thinking skills.

Each chapter includes:

- A list of the chapter **Key Terms**. Key terms appear in boldface type the first time they appear in your text, and are defined in the Glossary at the end of the textbook. (Definitions can also be found in a medical or standard dictionary.)
- **Chapter Review quiz questions**. Quiz questions reacquaint you with the material covered in your text and test your comprehension of the concepts presented.
- **Case Studies**. Additional case studies test your critical-thinking skills and your ability to apply the knowledge you've gained with a series of short-answer questions.
- **Concept Map Exercises**. This learning activity uses the concept maps in the textbook to help you master definitions and concepts. Concept maps can be considered a "web" of information. Individual terms have a tendency to get lost, but a web of interconnected terms is more easily maintained in memory.

Pathways to Student Success

Effective studying doesn't just happen. It involves carefully selecting and creating a suitable study site, putting yourself into the right frame of mind, being aware of your personal learning style, and some pretty basic study strategies.

SELECTING A STUDY AREA

To find the right study area, look for a distraction-free area where you can arrange your study materials properly. Make sure it has adequate lighting, is set at the right temperature, and is located among pleasant surroundings.

Before you begin to study, find a calm, comfortable place to study. As you select your study site, choose an area with the fewest distractions. After you find a study site you enjoy using, keep using it for subsequent study sessions. Using the same area creates familiarity and helps you begin studying as soon as you settle into the area.

Next, find the arrangement for studying you most enjoy. For most students, a desk with a comfortable, straight-backed chair makes the ideal study arrangement. You can arrange your study materials on the desk and easily reach them whenever necessary. Other students feel most comfortable in a large chair or sofa, with their books and other study materials spread out on the floor at their feet. A word of caution here: Don't get too relaxed. It's not a good idea to curl up on your bed to study; you're familiar with your bed as a sleeping place, and you may get sleepy. Sitting outside under a tree with a gentle breeze blowing might sound nice, but not when that gentle breeze becomes a distraction, ruffling papers in the wind. So choose your study arrangement carefully, weighing the value of the comfort it provides with its ability to meet your study needs.

To help you decide which study arrangement and study area are right for you, ask yourself these questions:

- Do I have sufficient work space?
- Can I keep the work space uncluttered?
- Do I have adequate lighting?
- Am I in a position that supports my back and eliminates muscle strain?
- Are there as few distractions as possible in the area?

Whichever study arrangement you choose, stay with it. Get into the habit of assuming your study position so you can get down to the business of studying quickly, with few distractions.

Lighting, temperature, and surroundings all play a part in creating a successful study site. Use either natural lighting or incandescent lighting for your study area, not fluorescent lighting. Your eyes are less likely to tire under direct light, like an incandescent lamp, than under indirect light. Keep the light from shining in your eyes by using overhead light or lighting from behind. The light should shine evenly on your work.

Choose a study area that's not too warm. Heat stress can decrease accuracy, speed, dexterity, and physical acuity. For most efficient studying, keep your study area cool—between 65°F and 70°F (18°C and 21°C).

Pleasant surroundings can greatly enhance study effectiveness. The sensations experienced while studying can be used later to trigger associations at test time. Pleasant surroundings also stimulate alertness. Minimize noise distractions while you study so you won't be disturbed. Turn your cell phone off or unplug the phone extension in your room. Leave the television off. You might also consider adding white noise to your environment. Instrumental music, the sound of a bubbling aquarium, and muted street sounds are examples of white noise. White noise helps cover distracting background sounds, such as the sounds of traffic or your roommate talking on the phone, and fills in periods of silence. In silence, even the sound of your own tapping pencil can be annoying.

Your physical comfort greatly affects your attitude about studying. When studying, make sure you assume a comfortable posture, use an appropriate reading angle, and move around periodically to enhance study effectiveness. Read while sitting in an upright position with your back straight or bent slightly forward. Other postures—particularly lying down—impair alertness and concentration. To decrease eyestrain, hold reading material at about a 45-degree angle from the flat surface of your desk or table to give you a clear view of the whole page. Reading material should also be kept at least 15 inches from your eyes. And remember to take a break about every hour to walk around, particularly if you need to ponder a point or repeat some facts to yourself. Walking around periodically when studying can enhance your brain's ability to learn new information and retain information. Do a few stretching exercises to get your circulation going and lessen muscle fatigue or tightness in your shoulders.

GETTING STARTED

One of the biggest challenges to effective studying is getting started. The first step in meeting that challenge is to break down large tasks into smaller ones. Several small tasks seem more achievable than one overwhelming one, and each smaller accomplishment provides moral support to finish the other tasks.

By taking small steps in the direction you want to go, you may end up at your destination sooner than you thought. For instance, you may not feel like reading your assignment, but if you tell yourself that you'll read for 5 minutes, at least you'll get a little reading done. After a few minutes, tell yourself that you'll read for a few more minutes, and so on. Pretty soon, you'll have read for a half hour or maybe even an hour and be well on your way to accomplishing—if not finishing—your assignment.

When beginning a study session, set a course for your studying or establish a purpose for it. Ask yourself, "What do I want to get out of this session? What do I need to know from the material?" After skimming the material, decide how deeply you need to become involved with the material. You may be responsible for detailed knowledge and intricate notes or you may need only a passing acquaintance with the material. Either way, plot your course before you start.

Remove the usual distractions—the telephone, television, and talk radio. Take care of your personal distractions, such as hunger or feeling hot. Schedule your study time so that it doesn't conflict with another activity you really want to do. Thinking about what you're missing can be a distraction in itself.

Find the right time to study, when you're feeling most efficient and receptive to information. Take a short break every hour to keep your study time energized. When concentration begins to lag, it's time for a break.

KNOW YOUR LEARNING STYLE

There are various styles of learning, including visual, auditory, and kinesthetic. If you know your learning style, you can structure your study sessions using the learning materials that most benefit your own personal learning style.

If you are an individual who learns best by watching how something is done or by reading about it, you are a visual learner. To make the most of this learning style, take advantage of all the visual information available to you, including such written and graphic information as books, handouts, demonstrations, Internet resources, personal notes, medical or scientific journals, periodicals, and videos. You can also make yourself flash cards or leave notes to yourself regarding difficult concepts on your bathroom mirror or the fridge. Tune into medical documentaries on television, or browse Internet medical sites for additional information.

If you learn best by hearing things, then you are an auditory learner. To make the most of this learning style, use as much auditory information as you can find. Dictate sample questions or questions from this Study Guide or the textbook into your own tape recorder and play them back in your car. Join (or start) a study group that meets regularly to share ideas and discuss concepts you're learning in class. Listen to audio books in the car or while you're traveling, or seek out an electronic medical dictionary that offers audio pronunciations of medical terms.

On the other hand, you're a kinesthetic learner if you prefer to jump right in and learn by doing. To make the most of this style of learning, take advantage of every opportunity to attend workshops, go on field trips, participate in group or class projects, tutor or teach others, or volunteer in a medical setting.

STUDY STRATEGIES

By using a number of study strategies you can give yourself the greatest chance to recall information later—on tests, quizzes, or even in a clinical setting. Using different strategies gives your brain more pathways to use when recalling information. Aside from setting up a good studying site and tuning in to your personal learning style, here are a few more tips for good study results.

- **Practice and repetition.** In learning, practice makes permanent! Practice helps the storage of information in long-term memory. Rehearsing is one method of practice. You can repeat information aloud or in a discussion, write or diagram the information repeatedly, or read and re-read information quietly several times. In general, speaking aloud or writing the information yield better results because they are more active processes, compared with the more passive practice of silent reading.
- **Spaced study.** Also known as "distributed practice," this method consists of alternating short study periods with breaks. Study goals are set by time (e.g., reading for at least 15 minutes) or task (reading a minimum of three pages). After reaching these goals, you can take a 5-minute to 15-minute break. This strategy works because it rewards your hard work, is completed in manageable portions of time, and it can keep you from confusing similar details when you have to study complex, interrelated information. And because the

work is completed under a deadline of time or task, your time spent studying is used more efficiently.

- **Interference reduction.** Interference happens when new information conflicts with background knowledge. For example, if you're trying to learn a lot of new terms, and two of the terms are similar, you might have trouble remembering either one of them. To avoid interference, try to relate new information to previously learned information—think about what makes the new information different from the older information.

- **Associations.** Forming acronyms or acrostics can help you recall lists of information. An acronym is a "word" created from the first letter of each item on a list. For example, Roy G. Biv is a popular acronym for the colors of the rainbow in order: red, orange, yellow, green, blue, indigo, violet. Acrostics are phrases or sentences represented on the vertical axis that are created from the first letter or letters of words in a list. For example, in music, an acrostic representing the lines on the treble clef is Every Good Boy Does Fine, which stands for the notes of the scale as they appear on the treble clef, from top to bottom: E, G, B, D, F. Acronyms and acrostics associate key information to an easily remembered word or phrase, thereby improving memory of the information.

- **Lists.** Lists help you organize ideas by categorizing the information according to some common theme. The arrangement of a list depends on your goals and the course emphasis and content. Recalling the name of the theme helps you remember the details of the items on that list.

- **Imagery.** The use of visual aids in studying can help you recall familiar and unfamiliar information. Imagery provides a different way of storing information, since visual images are stored differently in the brain than words. You can also use color as a visual aid by using various colors to highlight different types of information in your text or notebook, or adding doodles or symbols to your notes.

Learning from the World around You

The best way to learn about pathophysiology is to immerse yourself in the subject. Tell your friends and family what you are learning. Discover more about recent health advances from television, newspapers, magazines, and the Internet. Our knowledge about and understanding of the human body is constantly changing. The work you will do using this Study Guide can serve as a basis for lifelong learning about the functions and functional alterations of the human body.

Contents

Chapter 1

Introduction to Pathophysiology

KEY TERMS

acute	idiopathic	precipitating factors
asymptomatic	illness	prevalence
chronic	incidence	primary prevention
clinical manifestations	insidious	prognosis
concept	local	remission
diagnosis	morbidity	risk factors
disease	mortality	secondary prevention
endemic	multifactorial	signs
epidemic	nosocomial	structure
epidemiology	nursing diagnoses	subacute
etiology	pandemic	symptoms
exacerbation	pathogen	syndrome
function	pathogenesis	systemic
health	pathology	tertiary prevention
homeostasis	pathophysiology	
iatrogenic	physiology	

Chapter Review

1. In 2010, there was an outbreak of mumps in Iowa. A total of 604 cases were reported within just a few months. A dramatic increase of the number of cases of a disease within an area (such as a community or a state) is called a(n):

   a. Epidemic

   b. Pandemic

   c. Endemic

   d. Sociodemic

2. The avian flu is currently present in bird populations in many countries. At this time, the avian flu is not easily transmissible to humans. There is a concern, however, that the avian flu could mutate and become easily transmissible between humans. If this happens, and a large population of people is affected across the globe, it will be called a(n):

   a. Endemic

   b. Pandemic

   c. Epidemic

   d. Sociodemic

3. How does epidemiology contribute to the understanding of disease?

4. Observable signs and symptoms of the disease along with the clinical lab findings are called:

   a. Biochemical responses

   b. Clinical manifestations

   c. Congenital responses

   d. Developmental manifestations

5. Evidence of the alterations within the body as perceived by the patient are called:

   a. Lesions

   b. Injuries

   c. Symptoms

   d. Signs

6. List four or more human diversity factors that impact the variations in health and disease.

7. The process of assigning a name to a human response that is occurring in relation to an alteration within the body is called:

   a. Disease

   b. Nursing diagnosis

   c. Syndrome identification

   d. Etiology

8. René missed class this morning because she was ill. She has a fever, lethargy, generalized body aches, and a headache. Which of the following is not a systemic manifestation?

   a. Fever

   b. Lethargy

   c. Generalized body aches

   d. Headache

9. All of the following that René is experiencing are considered symptoms except:

   a. Fever

   b. Lethargy

   c. Generalized body aches

   d. Headache

10. Rhonda was infected with the varicella virus (chicken pox). This type of illness that develops quickly and does not last over an extended period of time is called a(n):

    a. Acute disease

    b. Chronic disease

    c. Etiology disease

    d. Iatrogenic disease

11. Ruby is a 33-year-old female. She was diagnosed with multiple sclerosis last year. Her health care provider told her that her disease progression would occur over a number of years and would most likely include periods of exacerbation and remission. This is an example of a(n) _____ disease.

    a. Acute

    b. Chronic

    c. Idiopathic

    d. Palliative

12. When Ruby experiences exacerbations of her multiple sclerosis, her symptoms:

    a. Disappear

    b. Flare and become severe

    c. Indicate remission of the disease

    d. Indicate a need for increased activity

13. Allen was diagnosed with pancreatic cancer. During the early stages of this disease, Allen was asymptomatic. This means that he:

    a. Was in remission

    b. Was in the idiopathic stage of the disease and did not experience symptoms

    c. Did not have any noticeable symptoms even though laboratory or other diagnostic tests may have indicated that the disease was present

    d. Experienced a nosocomial syndrome

14. The series of events that proceed from the cause of the disease to the development of clinical signs and symptoms is called _____ of the disease.

    a. The syndrome

    b. The pathogenesis

    c. The etiology

    d. The diagnosis

15. Compare and contrast the concepts of prevention versus intervention.

16. Jamie needed to have a catheter placed to decrease urinary retention while she was hospitalized. She proceeded to develop a urinary tract infection. The placement of the catheter contributed to this _____ illness.

    a. Unexpected

    b. Nosocomial

    c. Iatrogenic

    d. Unfortunate

17. Sam was recently diagnosed with lung cancer. He was told that it was probably caused by smoking along with his family history of lung cancer. What is the etiology of cancer in this case?

    a. Multifactorial

    b. Genetic

    c. Environmental

    d. Smoking

18. Stacy has had sinusitis now for 3 months. At this point, her sinusitis is considered:

    a. Acute

    b. Subacute

    c. Chronic

    d. Low-grade

19. John has asthma that gets worse with exercise. He needs to use an inhaler 10 to 15 minutes before gym class. The inhaler is designed to provide medication to relieve which type of clinical manifestations?

    a. Local

    b. Systemic

    c. Insidious

    d. Idiopathic

20. Go through the list of key terms. Define these as you go through the list. Write down the ones that you could not immediately define. Write the definitions and talk through what these terms mean with others in your class or your instructor.

Case Study 1.1

Aubre is a 48-year-old female. She lives on a farm in a rural community with her family. She has a history of type 2 diabetes and obesity. Aubre is also a past smoker, smoking approximately one pack per day for 20 years. She lives a very sedentary lifestyle and does not exercise routinely. One day while Aubre was making dinner, she noticed an aching pain in her shoulder. The pain increased in intensity to the point that she was unable to use her arm. Aubre made an appointment to see her physician early that afternoon. The physician diagnosed bursitis and treated her with oral anti-inflammatory medication.

Aubre returned home only to have the pain worsen. She returned to the clinic and saw the same physician. The physician injected her shoulder with cortisone (a steroid used for inflammation). Aubre returned home and the pain became so severe that she was incapacitated by it. Aubre's friend stopped by for a cup of coffee and found Aubre sitting slumped over in her chair. Aubre was pale, sweaty, and very nauseated. Aubre's friend called an ambulance to take her to the hospital. After being seen in the Emergency Department at the local hospital, Aubre was diagnosed as having an acute myocardial infarction (MI), or heart attack. The rural hospital was not able to care for her and she was transferred by ambulance to a larger hospital 60 miles away.

1. Describe one type of alteration you suspect that is oc curring in Aubre's body from the MI.

2. What are the lifestyle factors (risk factors) that may have had an impact on the development of the MI? Are the factors modifiable?

3. Did Aubre's gender potentially play a part in the delay of diagnosis and treatment of the MI? Discuss ways in which you could promote an individualized approach to the management of the diverse human response to illness.

Consider the alterations (e.g., alteration in tissue perfusion) that an MI might cause in the body and answer the following questions:

4. How is homeostasis disrupted because of this alteration?

5. How does the body attempt to compensate because of this alteration?

6. What human response (signs and symptoms) might you expect the patient to experience because of this alteration?

Concept Map Exercise

Drawing on what you have learned and studied in Chapter 1, fill in the missing terms in the concept map below.

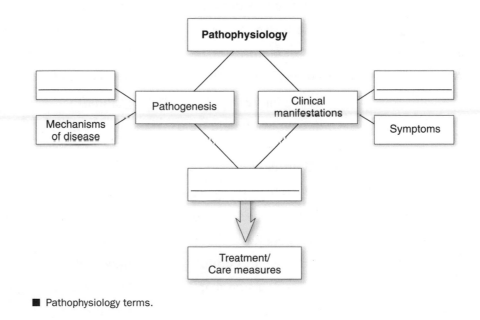

■ Pathophysiology terms.

Chapter 2

Altered Cells and Tissues

KEY TERMS

acromegaly

active transport

adaptation

adenoid hypertrophy

adenoma

adenosine triphosphate (ATP)

aerobic respiration

anaerobic respiration

antiport

apoptosis

atrophy

bilayer

binding affinity

bronchopulmonary dysplasia (BPD)

cardiac hypertrophy

cell

cerebral atrophy

chromatin

chromosomes

columnar epithelium

compliance

concentration gradient

cotransport

countertransport

cytoplasm

cytoskeleton

death

deficit injury

deoxyribonucleic acid (DNA)

differentiation

diffusion

dysplasia

ectocervix

endocervical canal

endocrine signaling

endocytosis

endogenous

endoplasmic reticulum

enzymes

epiphyseal

epithelium

exocytosis

exogenous

facilitated diffusion

feedback mechanism

free radical injury

genes

gigantism

glycolipid

glycolysis

golgi apparatus

hormones

human papilloma virus (HPV)

hydrophilic

hydrophobic

hypertrophy

hyperplasia

infection

ingest

insulin-like growth factor 1 (IGF-1)

integral protein

involution

ischemia

ligands

lipid bilayer

local mediators

lysosomes

mainstream smoke

malignancy

mechanical injury

membrane pore

membrane potential

menopause

metaplasia

mitochondria

mutations

necrosis

nucleus

nonpolar

oncogenic

organelles

organs

osmosis

osmotic pressure

oxygen free radicals

oxidative stress

paracrine signaling

passive smoke

peroxisomes

phagocytosis

phospholipids

physical injury

pinocytosis

plasma membrane

polar

primary active transport

proliferation

proteolysis

proteosomes

reactive oxygen species (ROS)

receptor

reproduction

respiration

secrete

secondary active transport

sidestream smoke

signal transduction pathway

spinal muscular atrophy

squamous epithelium

squamocolumnar junction

symport

syncope

syndactyly

thermal injury

tissue

transformation zone

transmembrane protein

trophic

Chapter Review

1. For the past 2 years, Sharon, a 54-year-old woman, has complained of mild burning in her chest after she eats. An upper GI endoscopy was performed and biopsies were taken from esophageal mucosa. The biopsies indicate the presence of columnar epithelium with goblet cells, which differ from the cells normally present in this area. Which of the following mucosal alterations is most likely represented by these findings?

   a. Dysplasia

   b. Hyperplasia

   c. Ischemia

   d. Metaplasia

2. Anne, a 25-year-old woman, gives birth to her second child and decides to breastfeed the baby. Which of the following cellular changes will occur within the breast?

   a. Dysplasia

   b. Atrophy

   c. Hyperplasia

   d. Metaplasia

3. Herbert, a 75-year-old male, died from left-sided heart failure. His heart had enlarged due to the increased workload due to the heart failure. The increased size of the heart is most likely due to which of the following processes involving the myocardial fibers?

   a. Fatty infiltration

   b. Hyperplasia

   c. Dysplasia

   d. Hypertrophy

4. Kate is a 13-year-old female who has come to have a left arm cast removed. She has had the cast on for 6 weeks. After the cast is removed, Kate expresses concern about the size of her left arm, stating that it appears much thinner than her right arm. You would tell her that this is most likely due to which of the following?

   a. Atrophy

   b. Dystrophy

   c. Anaplasia

   d. Dysplasia

5. Stephen, a 65-year-old male, suffered a myocardial infarction. During a myocardial infarction, the heart is deprived of oxygen and the cardiac cells suffer from ischemia. Cardiac cells that cannot adapt to the ischemia will suffer irreversible damage and die. This type of cell death is called:

   a. Necrosis

   b. Apoptosis

   c. Serotosis

   d. Cellular absorption

6. Characteristics of apoptosis include all of the following except:

   a. Referred to as "cellular suicide"

   b. Can be both a physiologic and pathologic cell response

    c. Occurs as a response to the removal of hormonal signals

    d. Is associated with inflammation

7. Acromegaly is a condition of:

    a. Hyperplasia

    b. Dysplasia

    c. Hypertrophy

    d. Anaplasia

8. John, a 44-year-old truck driver, has just been diagnosed with acromegaly. You would expect to see all of the following signs except:

    a. Soft tissue swelling

    b. Excessive increase in height

    c. Snoring

    d. Skin changes

9. John asks you to explain why this is occurring in his body. You tell him that:

    a. It is due to the nonfusion of his growth plates

    b. It is due to the hypersecretion of excessive growth hormone

    c. He is experiencing metaplasia due to the growth hormone

    d. It is a temporary response that will resolve in time

10. You are caring for Carolyn, a 16-year-old with human papilloma virus (HPV). Carolyn asks you what HPV is. You explain that it is a:

    a. Microbe

    b. Bacteria

    c. Virus

    d. Fungus

11. Carolyn states that she doesn't feel "sick" and wonders why there is a concern over the HPV. You know that:

    a. HPV isn't harmful and there is no need to be concerned

    b. The HPV will clear up on its own

    c. HPV is a benign flora of the cervix

    d. Some types of HPV are associated with the development of cervical cancer

12. Carolyn agrees to have the colposcopy procedure. She asks you what this procedure is involved with. You explain that all of the following occur except:

    a. Small punch biopsies are taken from the cervix and sent to pathology

    b. An instrument is used for visualization of the cervix

    c. The cervix is painted with an acetic acid solution

    d. The cervix is dilated for the procedure

13. The most significant change the pathologist will look for in the cells is:

    a. Dysplasia

    b. Hypertrophy

    c. Atrophy

    d. Metaplasia

14. Caryn is a smoker with a 12-year history of smoking a half-pack of cigarettes daily. She states that she feels fine and wonders why you suggest smoking cessation. You tell Caryn that cells respond to their environment. If the cell is exposed to a chronic irritation such as smoke or pollution, the cells in the airways will adapt. This change related to adaptation in the cells is called _____, which can lead to cancer.

    a. Hyperplasia

    b. Metaplasia

    c. Hypoplasia

    d. Dysplasia

15. Caryn is concerned about the threat of cancer. She asks if the cellular adaptation is reversible if she stops smoking now. You tell her that:

    a. No, the metaplasia will not be reversible

    b. Cells with metaplasia often return to their normal state when the irritation or stressor is removed

    c. The cells will not change any further, so there is no need for concern

    d. Metaplasia is a benign cellular adaptation

Case Study 2.1

Tom is a 39-year-old dairy farmer. Over the years, Tom has spent countless hours working in the sun. His wife had noticed an irregular-shaped dark mole on the inner aspect of his arm. She was concerned about the mole because of the color (variations of black and brown) and the irregular shape. She wanted Tom to make an appointment with their physician. Tom dismissed his wife's concern, stating that he felt fine. Tom stated that doctors are for sick people and he certainly did not feel sick. Besides, he stated, that he was too busy with the spring planting to spend time going to the clinic. Tom promised to go in at a later date when the work slowed down. When he was seen later that summer, the mole was removed and sent to the pathologist to determine if there were any irregularities of the cells in the tissue. Tom received a call from his provider and was informed that the mole was malignant melanoma, a type of skin cancer.

1. *Consider how health and illness relate to each other. Do you view the relationship as a static line with you moving between the two points?*

   Or do you perhaps view the relationship as a cycle, spending varying amounts of time in the states of health and illness?

   Considering how you relate the two concepts, identify your points of health and illness on the static line or the circle. That is, how far do you move away from "health" before you believe you are "ill"?

2. *Consider Tom's definition of health and illness. Where would he place himself on the continuum between health and illness? Where would* you *place him on the continuum? Why?*

3. *Envision the malignant melanoma cell. Draw a picture of it in the space below. Then draw healthy cells surrounding it. How might the malignant melanoma cell impose on the vital cell function of other healthy cells that surround it? How might it disrupt homeostasis within the body?*

4. *Consider the following cellular alterations: hypertrophy, hyperplasia, metaplasia, dysplasia, and atrophy. In the spaces below, draw each cell, and then identify any potential effects each cell might have on the surrounding normal cells.*

   Hypertrophy:

   Hypertrophy effects on surrounding normal cells:

   _____

   _____

Hyperplasia:

Hyperplasia effects on surrounding normal cells:

_____

_____

Metaplasia:

Metaplasia effects on surrounding normal cells:

_____

_____

Dysplasia:

Dysplasia effects on surrounding normal cells:

_____

_____

Atrophy:

Atrophy effects on surrounding normal cells:

_____

_____

5. *Which of the cellular alterations listed above are reversible? Why?*

Case Study 2.2

Joan is a 49-year-old married woman with four children. She works full time as the office manager in a small software company. During her routine yearly physical, you ask about her menstrual cycles. Joan tells you that she has noticed that they have become irregular with heavier bleeding at times. Her last menstrual period was 3 months ago. She also complains of vaginal dryness, fatigue, and mood swings. Joan asks you if she could possibly be entering menopause. She indicates concern about the changes her body is going through and wonders how this will affect her relationship with her husband. You explain that follicle stimulating hormone (FSH) stimulates the production of estrogen from the ovaries, so you will draw FSH and estradiol levels to better understand the cause of Joan's symptoms.

1. *What are the signs and symptoms associated with menopause?*

2. *What do you suspect Joan's FSH and estradiol blood levels will be? Why?*

3. *What is the alteration that is occurring in Joan's body? Why is this significant? How did Joan's body respond to this alteration?*

4. *In the space below, create a concept map of the structural and functional changes taking place within Joan's body during menopause. Next, add Joan's signs and symptoms to the concept map. Connect the signs and symptoms with the structural and functional changes taking place.*

5. *Consider Joan's concern about how menopause will affect her relationship with her husband. How would you respond?*

ACTIVITY: COMPLETE THE CROSSWORD PUZZLE USING THE FOLLOWING CLUES:

Across

1. Relating to disease, the observable or measurable expression of the altered health condition

4. An indicator that is reported by an ill individual and is often considered a "subjective" manifestation

9. _____ factors: vulnerabilities that, when present, increase the chances that a disease may occur

10. Groups of similar cell types that combine to perform a specific function

11. The rate of occurrence of a health condition at any given time

12. The type of blood vessel that carries blood to the heart

13. Describes manifestations or illnesses that are often more insidious and generally last 6 months or longer

14. Changing of one cell type to another

17. Cellular structures must _____ their function when faced with damage and injury for the cell to survive.

18. Cellular respiration uses _____ to oxidize fuel molecules and results in the production of energy.

21. The smallest component of the living individual

24. The cause of the disease

26. _____ injury: damage caused by extremes of temperature

28. Decrease in the size of the cell

29. The reactions of the body to forces of a deleterious nature that disturb homeostasis

31. The system within an organism that protects against infection by identifying and killing pathogens

32. Movement of water across a concentration gradient

33. _____ apparatus: cellular organelle with a membranous structure; prepares substances produced by the endoplasmic reticulum for secretion out of the cell

Down

2. Describes illnesses that are the inadvertent result of medical treatment

3. Describes illnesses that are caused by exposure to the health care system

4. Estrogen is an example of a _____ hormone.

5. Adenosine triphosphate (ATP)–requiring process of ingesting very small vesicles

6. The percentage of a population that is affected by a particular disease at a given time

7. The largest organ of the integumentary system made up of multiple layers of epithelial tissues

8. Acronym for the nucleic acid that contains a sugar (ribose); responsible for control of protein synthesis

15. A state of inadequate blood flow to peripheral tissues

16. Programmed cell death that is prompted by a genetic signal and designed to replace old cells with new; also known as "cellular suicide"

19. The symptoms of acromegaly are related to excessive _____.

20. Disorderly process of cell death associated with inflammation

22. Biologic catalysts that accelerate the speed of chemical reactions in the body

23. Refers to those manifestations that are directly at the site of injury, or infection and are confined to a specific site

25. Clinical manifestations of acromegaly include coarse _____ growth.

27. Acronym for the toxic oxygen molecules or radicals that are formed by the reaction between oxygen and water during mitochondrial respiration

30. Acronym for a medical test that evaluates electrical activity of the heart

Chapter 3

Inflammation and Tissue Repair

KEY TERMS

abscess

adherence

adhesions

angiogenesis

ankylosis

arachidonic acid

arthritis

autoimmunity

basement membrane

basophil

cardinal signs

cellular response

chemotactic factors

chemotaxis

collagen

contractures

cytokines

debridement

deep partial-thickness burns

degranulation

dehiscence

diapedesis

differentiation

dilate

dyspepsia

elastin

endothelial cells

epithelioid cells

erythema

eschar

extracellular matrix

exudate

fibroblasts

fistula

friability

full-thickness burns

gastritis

giant cells

glycoproteins

granulation tissue

granuloma

immune response

inflammatory mediators

injury

keloids

labile cells

leukocytosis

lymphadenitis

lysis

mast cell

occult

opsonization

pannus

parenchymal

perfusion

permanent cells

permeable

phagocytosis

platelet-activating
   factor

primary intention

proliferation

proteinases

provisional matrix

pyrexia

re-epithelialization

regeneration

resolution

secondary intention

sepsis

serous exudate

shock

stable cells

superficial partial-
   thickness burns

thrombus

ulcers

vascular response

Chapter Review

1. Acute inflammation occurs in response to:

   a. Cellular repair

   b. Tissue injury

   c. Scar formation

   d. Cellular reproduction

2. Inflammation is a process that includes the following:

   a. Vascular and cellular responses

   b. The formation of exudates

   c. Preparation for tissue repair

   d. a and c

   e. a, b, and c

3. The preferred outcome from the inflammation process is:

   a. Tissue repair or regeneration

   b. Cellular alteration with scar tissue formation

   c. Metaplasia

   d. Cellular hypertrophy

4. You are caring for Andrew, a 5-year-old boy in the emergency department. He has a sliver in his right index finger that has been present for 2 days. Andrew refused to let his mother remove the sliver and now the tissue around the sliver is red, warm, and swollen. What is the most likely cause of the warmth and swelling?

a. The release of prostaglandins

b. Cytokines

c. Vasoconstriction in the microcirculation

d. Increased blood flow to the area due to vasodilation

5. You know that the most important roles for chemical mediators are to:

a. Release histamine

b. Constrict vessels to control potential bacterial invasion in the area

c. Induce vasodilation and increase capillary permeability

d. Cause pain in order to decrease mobility

6. During the inflammation process, the vascular response triggers the following changes at the site of the injury except:

a. Vasodilation

b. Increased permeability of vessels

c. Vasoconstriction

d. Increased blood flow

7. In order for the cellular response to occur, which of the following processes need to take place?

a. Cellular migration

b. Cellular adherence

c. Chemotaxis

d. a and b

e. a, b, and c

8. The inflammation process must prepare the site of injury for healing. This includes cleaning up the debris (dead and impaired tissue) at the site. This process of engulfing and digesting impaired tissue is called:

a. Chemotaxis

b. Diapedesis

c. Phagocytosis

d. Degranualtion

9. Cells that play a role in phagocytosis include:

a. Neutrophils

b. Monocytes

c. Macrophages

d. All of the above

10. Which of the following best describes the inflammatory process in relation to an acute injury?

    a. Increased vascular permeability, dilation of vessels, and leukocyte attraction to the site of the injury

    b. Release of chemical mediators and vessel constriction

    c. Vessels dilate causing the release of chemical mediators

    d. None of the above

11. The primary signs and symptoms of acute inflammation include all of the following except:

    a. Redness and heat

    b. Swelling

    c. Pain and loss of function

    d. a and c

    e. All of the above

12. During the inflammation process, a fever would be an example of:

    a. A local response to the inflammation process

    b. A systemic response to the inflammation process

    c. An indirect action

    d. A holistic response

13. Katelynn, a 13-year-old female, is accompanied to the emergency department by her mother. Katelynn hit a tree with her four-wheeler and has large abrasions on her right knee and forehead. Her mother asks if Katelynn will need "stitches." You know that this type of wound will most likely heal by:

    a. Primary intention

    b. Secondary intention

    c. Leukocyte adherence

    d. Third intention

14. Katelynn asks what she can do to help the abrasions heal faster. All of the following are important factors in wound healing except:

    a. Integrity of the vascular and cellular inflammatory responses

    b. Reformation of the extracellular matrix

    c. Regeneration of those cells capable of mitosis

    d. Decreased protein synthesis

15. Chronic inflammation differs from acute inflammation because it:

    a. Triggers the cellular response before the vascular response

    b. Occurs for a period of 1 week after the acute stage of inflammation

    c. Involves different cells

    d. Represents a persistent or recurrent state of inflammation lasting several weeks or longer

16. Ulcerative colitis is found in the:

    a. Large intestine

    b. Small intestine

    c. Stomach

    d. Anywhere in the GI tract from the mouth to anus

17. A major difference between Crohn disease and ulcerative colitis is the presence of ____ in Crohn disease.

    a. A chronic inflammatory response

    b. Ulcers

    c. Skip lesions

    d. Histamine

18. A patient is diagnosed with ulcerative colitis. She has more than four bowel movements per day but no fever, weakness, fatigue, or other systemic manifestations. Her disease would be classified as:

    a. Mild

    b. Moderate

    c. Severe

    d. In remission

19. A patient is diagnosed with achilles tendonitis. What would you expect to be the clinical manifestations of this condition given what you know about acute inflammation?

    a. Heel pain, swelling, limited range of motion

    b. Fever, anorexia, weakness

    c. Redness, inability to walk, ankylosis

    d. Fibrosis, degeneration, scarring

20. A major aspect of treatment for inflammatory conditions is:

    a. Ice, rest, elevation, compression

    b. Removal of the source of injury when possible

c. Acetaminophen (Tylenol)

d. Use of steroids

Case Study 3.1

Brian is an active 13-year-old boy who lives on a farm. During the spring planting season, he was filling the tractor with fuel. As he was taking the nozzle out of the tank, a spark ignited the fuel. Brian dropped the nozzle and ran to the house. His elder sister pushed him to the ground and smothered the flames on his shirt. Brian was taken to the emergency department for the treatment of his burns. He had deep partial-thickness burns covering both of his arms.

1. *Consider the inflammatory response in relation to Brian's burns. What kinds of local and systemic responses are occurring both at the site of injury and within Brian's body? What is triggering these responses?*

2. *Would you expect Brian to experience pain with this type of burn? Why or why not?*

3. *What clinical manifestations would you expect to see with Brian's injury? Why are you seeing these particular manifestations (what processes are occurring within the body that are causing these manifestations)? Draw a map that links the manifestations to the causes.*

4. *Consider the healing process that takes place with this type of injury. How is new tissue formed?*

5. *Discuss different types of treatment options available for Brian.*

6. *Discuss the potential complications of this type of burn in relation to the following:*

   a. *A widespread inflammatory response*

   b.   *Stress hypermetabolism*

   c.   *Impaired defense mechanisms*

Case Study 3.2

Terri is a 42-year-old female. She is married and has four children. Terri lives a very active lifestyle and enjoys gardening and sewing. She recently saw her health care provider because she had pain in her hands. The pain was limiting the activities that Terri could participate in. Terri also noted that the joints in her fingers were erythematous and that she felt very tired most of the time. Terri was diagnosed with rheumatoid arthritis. She was referred to a rheumatologist for treatment.

1. *Rheumatoid arthritis is an example of chronic inflammation. Compare and contrast the process of acute inflammation and the process of chronic inflammation.*

2. *Discuss the cellular response and adaptation to the chronic inflammation that is occurring within Terri's joints.*

3. *Draw a concept map linking the cellular response and adaptation to the long-term alterations Terri will experience with rheumatoid arthritis. Do these alterations have any impact on other tissue/systems within the body?*

4. *Describe the structural and functional changes that occur as a result of rheumatoid arthritis.*

5. *How will Terri's body attempt to compensate for these changes?*

6. *Consider this: How would having rheumatoid arthritis change your current lifestyle?*

Concept Map Exercises

Drawing on what you have learned and studied in Chapter 3 about the body's response to injury, tissue repair, chemical mediators, and inflammation, fill in the missing terms in the concept maps below.

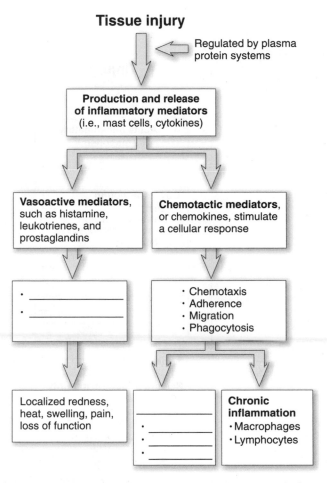

■ An overview of the importance of chemical mediators in the vascular and cellular responses of inflammation. (Image modified from Rubin E, Farber JL. *Pathology*. 4th ed. Philadelphia: Lippincott Williams & Wilkins; 2005, with permission.)

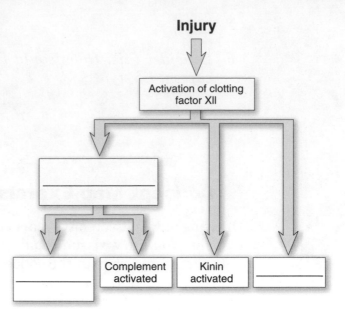

■ An example of one mechanism of the interrelationship between the clotting, complement, and kinin systems: activation of clotting factor XII.

Injury

Activation of clotting factor XII

Complement activated

Kinin activated

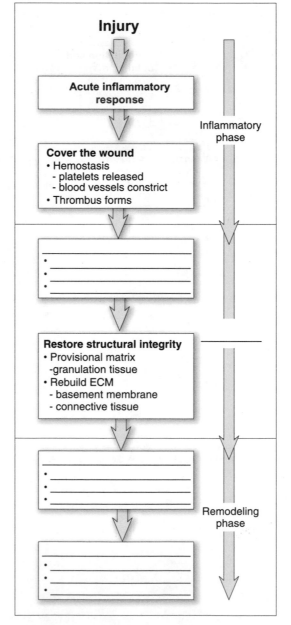

■ Phases of healing and tissue repair.

Injury

Acute inflammatory response

Cover the wound
• Hemostasis
 - platelets released
 - blood vessels constrict
• Thrombus forms

Restore structural integrity
• Provisional matrix
 -granulation tissue
• Rebuild ECM
 - basement membrane
 - connective tissue

Inflammatory phase

Remodeling phase

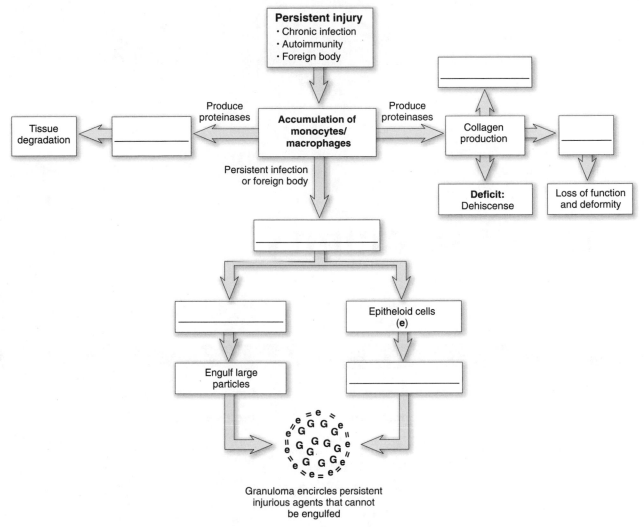

Persistent injury
· Chronic infection
· Autoimmunity
· Foreign body

Produce
proteinases

**Accumulation of
monocytes/
macrophages**

Produce
proteinases

Tissue
degradation

_____

Collagen
production

_____

Persistent infection
or foreign body

Deficit:
Dehiscense

Loss of function
and deformity

_____

_____

Epitheloid cells
(e)

Engulf large
particles

_____

Granuloma encircles persistent
injurious agents that cannot
be engulfed

■ The process of chronic inflammation leading to granuloma formation.

Chapter 4

Altered Immunity

KEY TERMS

adaptive immunity

adjuvant

allergens

alloantibodies

alloantigens

allograft

amniocentesis

anaphylaxis

angioedema

antibodies

antigen

antigen-presenting cells

antigenic variation

Arthus reaction

atopic

attenuated

autograft

autoimmune

B cell receptor

B lymphocytes

basophils

blood transfusion

blood typing

bronchospasm

CD4 T lymphocytes

CD8 T lymphocytes

Cell-mediated immunity

cellular casts

clonal expansion

clonal selection

clusters of differentiation

conjugated vaccines

constant region

cortisol

cross matching

cytotoxic T lymphocytes

delayed hypersensitivity reactions

dendritic cells

direct cell-mediated toxicity

discoid

effector cells

elicitation phase

eosinophils

familial tendency

graft versus host disease (GVHD)

granulocytes

helper T lymphocytes

hematopoietic stem cells

hemolytic

host

human immunodeficiency virus (HIV)

human leukocyte antigens (HLAs)

humoral immunity

hyperacute graft rejection

IgE

immunity

immunodeficiency

immunoglobulins (Ig)

immunologic memory

immunology

innate immunity

Langerhans' cells

Latencylymphadenopathy

lymphatic ignorance

lymphatic system

lymph fluid

lymph nodes

lymphoid progenitor

macrophage

major histocompatibility complex (MHC)

major histocompatibility complex class I (MHC I)

major histocompatibility complex class II (MHC II)

malar

memory cells

molecular mimicry

monocytes

myeloid progenitor

naive lymphocytes

natural killer cells

neutralization

neutrophil

nonself

opsonization

pericarditis

peripheral organs

photosensitivity

placenta

pleuritis

polygenic

polymorphic

proteinuria

quiescence

regulatory T cells

sensitization phase

seroconversion

suppressor T lymphocytes

supraphysiologic

T cell receptor

T_H1

T_H2

T lymphocytes

thrombocytopenia

transcription

ulcers

urticaria

vaccines

variable regions

viscosity

Chapter Review

1. Rita is a 20-year-old college student. She leads a very active lifestyle and belongs to the Hiking Club at school. Rita and a group of friends had planned an overnight hike in the desert. During their first day out, Rita was bitten by a snake. She was transported to the nearest hospital. As part of her treatment, Rita was given gamma globulin. Rita asks why they gave her this. You explain that the gamma globulin promotes:

   a. Acquired active immunity

   b. Naturally acquired passive immunity

   c. Artificially acquired active immunity

   d. Artificially acquired passive immunity

2. John has developed an allergy to bee stings. Which immunoglobulin is activated during his body's response to a bee sting?

   a. IgG

   b. IgA

   c. IgM

   d. IgE

3. John's body has an exaggerated response to a bee sting. This response would be defined as:

   a. Autoimmunity

   b. Hypersensitivity

   c. Alloimmunity

   d. Failure of host defense mechanisms

4. Your friend Sharilee is entering the nursing major at your college. As part of the admission requirements, she needs to have the hepatitis B vaccination. Sharilee asks you why she needs to have this vaccination. You tell her that it promotes the following type of immunity:

   a. Naturally acquired active immunity

   b. Naturally acquired passive immunity

   c. Artificially acquired active immunity

   d. Artificially acquired passive immunity

5. Your friend Mona has a 4-year-old sister named Tyra. She tells you that over the weekend the mother of one of Tyra's friends called to say that her daughter had the chicken pox (varicella-zoster virus). If Tyra develops chicken pox, what type of immunity will she develop?

   a. Naturally acquired active immunity

   b. Naturally acquired passive immunity

   c. Artificially acquired active immunity

   d. Artificially acquired passive immunity

6. Mona then asks you how the antibodies that Tyra develops will protect her from future encounters with the varicella-zoster virus. You tell her that antibodies protect the body in all of the following ways except:

   a. Assist with the binding of the antigen to the antibody

   b. Help promote phagocytosis and destruction of the pathogen

   c. Assist with activation of complement

   d. Help to bind the neutrophils to the T cells

7. Live microbes that have been modified with reduced virulence for incorporation into vaccines are referred to as being _____.

   a. Immune toxoids

   b. Attenuated

   c. Killed

   d. Compliment activated

8. Ty has leukemia. Because of the leukemia, his immune system suffers from an alteration called immunosuppression. Which of the following immunizations would carry the greatest risk for this type of patient?

   a. Immune serums

   b. Toxoids

   c. Attenuated vaccines

   d. Killed, inactivated vaccines

9. Which of the following is true about innate immunity?

   a. It is highly effective against many virus infections

   b. It is highly specific and adaptive

   c. It is the first to respond to pathogen challenge

   d. It is slower to respond than adaptive immunity

10. Your neighbor is pregnant with her first child. She tells you that she needs to receive a RhIg injection. She understands why she must receive the injection but does not understand how the RhIg works. You tell her that the RhIg attaches to the:

    a. White blood cells

    b. Antigen in the mother's blood

    c. Antigen in the baby's blood

    d. Antibody in the mother's blood

11. Major characteristics related to the adaptive immune system include all of the following except:

    a. Specificity and diversity

    b. Memory

    c. Antigen replacement

    d. Self and non-self recognition

12. Cell-mediated immunity protects the body in all of the following ways except:

    a. It decreases antibody production

    b. It activates macrophages

    c. It activates antigen specific cytotoxic T lymphocytes

    d. It stimulates the production of cytokines

13. These cells display antigens for recognition by the cytotoxic T lymphocytes:

    a. T helper lymphocytes

    b. Neutrophils

    c. Granulocytes

    d. Eosinophils

14. Alteration within the immune system can result from all of the following except:

    a. Failure of host defense mechanisms

    b. IgM immune memory

    c. Hypersensitivity

    d. Autoimmunity and alloimmunity

15. Examples of a type II antibody-mediated reaction include all of the following except:

    a. Blood transfusion reactions

    b. Graves' disease

    c. Hemolytic disease of the newborn

    d. Systemic lupus erythematosus

Case Study 4.1

Andrea is 35 years old. She is a nurse and works in a long-term care center. She is at the clinic today because she has concerns about some symptoms that she has been experiencing for the past couple of years. She states that she is very sensitive to the sun. You note that Andrea has a rash on her cheeks. Andrea also complains of pain in her joints of her fingers as well as fatigue. You note that her joints are red and swollen. The primary health care provider orders the following tests: antinuclear antibodies and antidouble stranded DNA. Andrea is diagnosed with systemic lupus erythematosus (SLE).

1. Describe the alteration occurring within Andrea's immune system.

2. What clinical manifestations does Andrea have? List each manifestation and then discuss its relationship to the alterations that are occurring within her immune system.

3. Define the importance of the recognition of the body's "self" antigens from foreign "non-self" antigens in relation to SLE.

4. List the major treatments for SLE. How is each treatment targeting the alteration within the body?

Case Study 4.2

Trish is a single 20-year-old college student. She comes into the college health center because she has been very tired lately. Trish also complains of being sick all of the time stating, "I catch cold after cold and can't seem to get over one before I get another." Trish also appears very stressed and tells you that her boyfriend that she has been in a relationship with for the past 6 months told her that he had tested positive for HIV. Trish is concerned that she may also be infected with the virus.

1. Discuss the alterations that occur within the immune system with HIV and AIDS. What parts of the immune system are affected?

2. Discuss the relationship of the clinical manifestations to the alterations that are occurring in her immune system.

3. How does the body respond to the alterations that occur within the immune system affected by AIDS?

4. What treatments are available for HIV and AIDS?

◢ **Concept Map Exercises**

Drawing on what you have learned and studied in Chapter 4, fill in the missing terms in the concept map below.

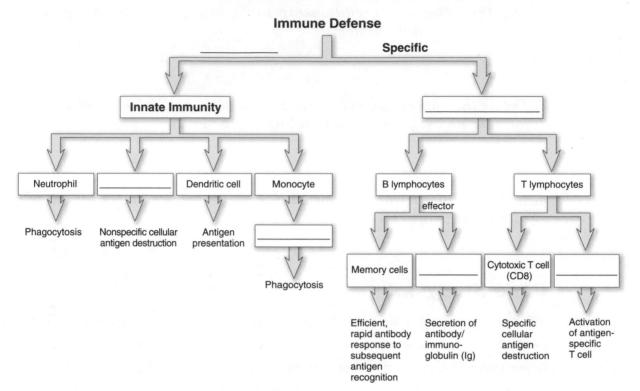

■ Concept map. Cellular components involved in immune defense.

Chapter 5

Infection

KEY TERMS

acute clinical illness
aerobic
airborne transmission
anaerobic
antigenic variability
antigenicity
ascending
autoclave
bacteremia
bacteria
Brudzinski sign
cirrhosis
coinfection
communicable
convalescence
cytosol
dermatophyte
direct contact
droplet transmission
dysuria
endotoxin
erythropoiesis
exotoxins
exposure
facultative parasites

fulminant hepatitis
hematuria
host
hyphae
icteric phase
icterus
incubation
infectivity
jaundice
Kernig sign
Kupffer cells
latency
leukocytosis
leukopenia
maceration
molds
mycelium
mycoses
nuchal rigidity
obligate parasites
opportunistic pathogens
pathogen
pathogenic defense
    mechanisms
pathogenicity

photophobia
portal circulation
prodrome
pseudohyphae
purulent
pyelonephritis
pyogenic
pyuria
reassortment
recovery
resident flora
septic shock
septicemia
superinfection
toxigenicity
universal precautions
urgency
vector
vector transmission
virions
virulence
viruses
yeasts

Chapter Review

1. Tissue destruction that is the result of the invasion of microorganisms is called:

   a. Resident flora intervention

   b. Pathogen destruction

   c. Receptor binding

   d. Infectious disease

2. *Escherichia coli* is present within the gastrointestinal tract and does not pose any harm to the body. This type of bacteria is an example of:

   a. Resident flora

   b. Anaerobic flora

   c. An overproliferation of bacteria

   d. A fungal infection

3. Caren is a 22-year-old female. She comes into the clinic because she suspects that she has a urinary tract infection. Most urinary tract infections are caused by the bacteria *Escherichia coli*. When *E. coli* moves into another part of the body where it is not normally present and causes problems it is called a:

   a. Host cell

   b. Receptor

   c. Pathogen

   d. Parasite

4. Alexia has had a cold for the past week. During school she coughs and sneezes. One of her friends, Donna, also becomes infected with the virus and develops symptoms 1 week later. When considering the chain of infection, the coughing and sneezing was most likely the:

   a. Vector

   b. Mode of transmission

   c. Reservoir

   d. Portal of entry

5. Donna's exposure to the cold virus occurred when she was with Alexia. However, Donna did not experience symptoms of a cold right away. This period of time from the time of exposure until Donna developed symptoms is called the:

   a. Incubation period

   b. Exposure period

   c. Prodromal period

   d. Convalescence period

6. Teri's brother accidentally hooked her arm with a fish hook while they were fishing for sunfish off of their grandparents' dock. Her grandfather removed the hook and cleansed the area with soap and water. One week later, an infection developed and the tissue around the wound was red, painful, swollen, and warm to touch. The redness, pain, swelling, and warmth in the tissue are due to the:

   a. Inflammation process

   b. Bactericidal process

   c. Septic shock

   d. Chronic infection

7. Teri's mom took her into the clinic to see their health care provider. The provider prescribed an antibacterial medication for Teri to take. Teri doesn't understand how a pill that she takes is going to help the infection in her arm. Teri is told that an antibacterial medication works because it does all of the following except:

   a. Inhibits synthesis of the bacteria cell wall

   b. Damages the cytoplasmic membrane of the bacteria

   c. Disables nucleic acid metabolism or protein synthesis

   d. Promotes bacterial cell wall enlargement

8. The redness, warmth, and swelling around the site of injury in Teri's arm are considered:

   a. Systemic signs of infection

   b. Local signs of infection

   c. Septicemia

   d. Chronic infection

9. Besides the antibacterial medication that Teri was given, her health care provider also encouraged her to rest, take in plenty of oral fluids, and use acetaminophen for the pain. These types of treatments are called:

   a. Fungicidal treatment

   b. Prodromal treatment

   c. Symptomatic treatment

   d. Bactericidal treatment

10. Influenza is a virus that has the ability to change and adapt to its host. This ability to change genetic composition during replication in the human host cell is called:

    a. Host adaptation

    b. Reassortment

    c. Realignment

    d. Prodromal communication

11. The portal of entry into the human host for the influenza virus is the:

    a. Skin

    b. Mucous membrane

    c. Gastrointestinal tract

    d. Respiratory tract

12. Ellen, your neighbor, has contracted the influenza virus. She knows that you are taking pathophysiology and asks you how a simple virus can cause her sore throat, cough, and nasal congestion. You explain that the localized clinical manifestations that someone with influenza experiences are caused by:

    a. A septic response

    b. The inflammatory response and cell death

    c. The virus separation mode

    d. Nucleic acid metabolism

13. Shana has scheduled a visit with a fertility clinic because she is unable to become pregnant. When taking her history, it is noted that she had been diagnosed with numerous sexually transmitted infections in the past. Shana wonders how those infections in the past could possibly affect her ability to become pregnant now. You know that repeated or chronic infections will:

    a. Result in scar tissue formation within the fallopian tubes

    b. Enhance ovulation

c. Decrease the risk for future sexually transmitted infections

d. Increase the number of eggs released from the fallopian tubes

14. Amy is a 3-month-old baby who has been hospitalized because of meningitis. Her treatment includes IV antibiotic therapy. After the therapy has started, her health status begins to decline quickly. You understand that the bacteria that causes meningitis is gram-negative. Considering this, Amy's decline in health status is most likely due to the fact that:

a. The gram-negative bacteria react with gram-positive bacteria

b. The bacteria are not killed by the antibiotic

c. As the bacteria were killed, endotoxins within the cell wall were released and they triggered a massive inflammatory response

d. The bacteria are causing a hypersensitivity response

15. An 80-year-old grandmother is admitted to the hospital for a hip fracture. During her stay on the orthopaedic unit, she develops an infection in her surgical wound. This type of infection that develops while a patient is in a hospital is called a(n):

a. Chronic infection

b. Nosocomial infection

c. Ascending infection

d. Recurrent infection

16. Debbie develops a yeast infection. During the health history, she is asked if she has recently been on antibiotics. Debbie wonders what this has to do with yeast. The practitioner explains:

a. Yeasts are destroyed by antibiotics

b. Yeasts grow best when the patient is febrile

c. Yeasts do not have to compete with resident bacteria and can overgrow

d. The question was unrelated to her current concern

17. Which of the following helps to explain why certain populations become infected by certain pathogens and others do not?

a. Average age of the population

b. Viral reassortment

c. Direct destruction

d. Receptor binding

18. Which of the following is *not* a mechanism by which pathogens cause disease?

    a. Direct destruction of the host cell

    b. Cellular restoration

    c. Interference with host cell's metabolic function

    d. Exposure to toxins

19. Which of the following terms relates to potency, and therefore the pathogen's ability to cause disease, in large populations even with minimal exposure?

    a. Virulence

    b. Antigenicity

    c. Infectivity

    d. Toxigenicity

20. Tom goes to the clinic for sexually transmitted infection (STI) testing. He is told that he has chlamydia and gonorrhea. The health care practitioner indicates that this is a common _____.

    a. Chronic infection

    b. Coinfection

    c. Superinfection

    d. Recurrent infection

21. What is the difference between obligate and facultative parasites?

    a. Obligate can live independently of the host

    b. Facultative can live independently of the host

    c. Facultative are capable of producing exotoxins

    d. Obligate are much smaller in size than facultative

22. Which pathogen is not known to elicit a notable immune response?

    a. Bacteria

    b. Viruses

    c. Prions

    d. Parasites

23. Becky has an infection and her white blood cell count indicates leukopenia. Which of the following is most likely to be occurring?

    a. Viral infection

    b. Bacterial infection

    c. Fungal infection

    d. Adequate immune response

24. Which of the following is a major meningitis risk factor for college students?

    a. Homework

    b. Living in close quarters in dormatories or apartments

    c. Athletic competition

    d. Poor nutritional intake

25. What nutrition teaching would be included for the patient with viral hepatitis and impaired bile production?

    a. High protein diet

    b. Low fat diet

    c. Low carbohydrate diet

    d. High fiber diet

Case Study 5.1

Martha is an 80-year-old female who lives alone in her apartment. Martha became ill and demonstrated the following signs and symptoms: sore throat, nasal congestion, and drainage. Martha also complained of experiencing chills, fever, body aches, weakness, and malaise. Martha's daughter brought her in to see her health care provider. During the visit, a chest X-ray and rapid viral assay test were ordered. The findings on the chest X-ray were indicative of pneumonia and the rapid viral assay test was positive for influenza. Martha states that she cannot have influenza as she received a "flu shot" 2 years ago. In fact, she was going out of her way to help care for others in her apartment building who had influenza because she felt she was protected with her "flu shot."

1. *What type of organism causes influenza? How does this impact the lungs? Describe the normal mechanisms in place that protect against infection.*

2. *Is it possible for Martha to have contracted the influenza virus even though she had a "flu shot" 2 years ago? Why or why not?*

3. *Why did so many elderly have the influenza virus in Martha's apartment building?*

4. *How could you help Martha decrease her risk of contracting the virus next flu season?*

5. *Draw a concept map of the chain of infection; identify how to break the chain of influenza at each of the points: reservoir, portal of exit, route of transmission, portal of entry, host factors.*

▨ **Concept Map Exercises**

Drawing on what you have learned and studied in Chapter 5, fill in the missing terms in the concept maps below.

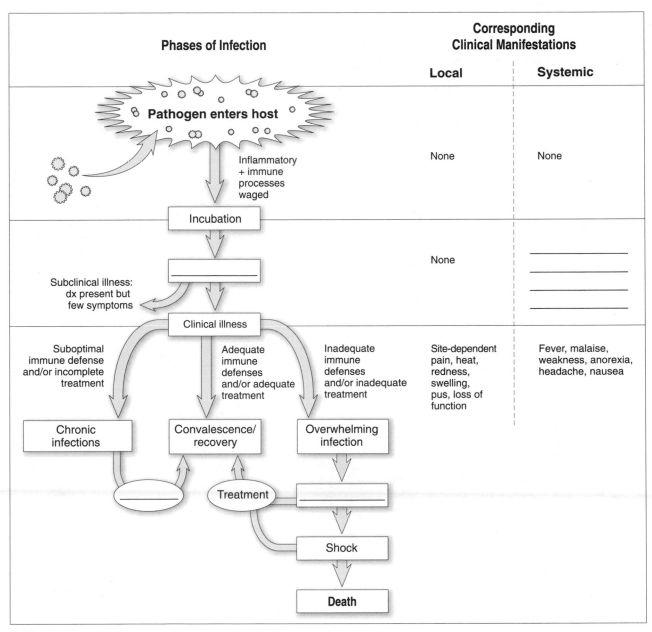

Phases of Infection

Corresponding Clinical Manifestations

	Local	Systemic
Pathogen enters host	None	None
Inflammatory + immune processes waged		
Incubation	None	_____ _____ _____ _____
Subclinical illness: dx present but few symptoms		
Clinical illness	Site-dependent pain, heat, redness, swelling, pus, loss of function	Fever, malaise, weakness, anorexia, headache, nausea

Suboptimal immune defense and/or incomplete treatment

Adequate immune defenses and/or adequate treatment

Inadequate immune defenses and/or inadequate treatment

Chronic infections

Convalescence/ recovery

Overwhelming infection

Treatment

Shock

Death

■ Phases of infection and corresponding clinical manifestations.

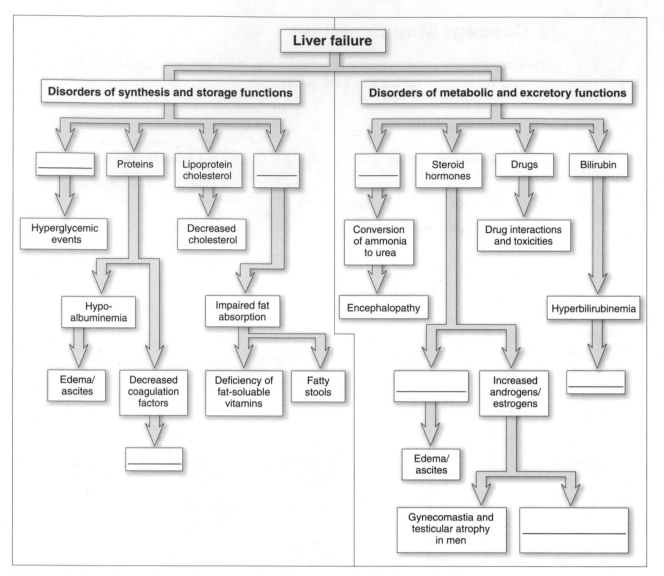

■ Alterations in liver function and manifestations of liver failure. (Image modified from Porth CM. *Pathophysiology: Concepts of Altered Health States*. 7th ed. Philadelphia: Lippincott Williams & Wilkins; 2004.)

◤ Activity: A Comparison of Common Pathogens

Complete the table below.

Pathogen	Unique Structure Characteristics	Replication	Toxin Production	Treatment Measures
Bacteria				
Viruses				
Prions				
Fungi				
Protozoa				

Chapter 6

Genetic and Developmental Disorders

allele

alternative splicing

amino acids

aneuploidy

autosomes

base pairs

bilirubin

blastomere

carriers

centromere

chromosomes

codon

congenital defects

cytochrome oxidase (COX)

deoxyribonucleic acid (DNA)

diploid

dominant

dyskinesia

epigenetic

exon

expressivity

fetal alcohol syndrome (FAS)

gamete

genetic code

genomic imprinting

genomics

genotype

haploid

hemoglobin A (HbA)

hemoglobin S (HbS)

hemolysis

heredity

heterozygous

heteroplasmy

homozygous

hygroma

intron

karyotype

matrilineal

messenger RNA (mRNA)

meiosis

Mendelian pattern of inheritance

mitosis

monosomy

mosaicism

mutations

nondisjunction

nuchal translucency

organogenesis

penetrance

phenotype

polygenic

polymorphism

preimplantation genetic diagnosis

purine

pyrimidine

quadruple test

recessive

ribonucleic acid (RNA)

ribosomal RNA (rRNA)

sex chromosome

sex-linked

short tandem repeats (STR)

sickle cell anemia	teratogen	translocation
sickle cell trait	transfer RNA (tRNA)	translucency
single gene trait	transcription	trisomy
somatic mutation	translation	

Chapter Review

1. The information within the genes that contain the directions for making a specific protein is called:

   a. Genetic code

   b. Base pairs

   c. Pyrimidines

   d. Introns

2. Which of the following transcribes the DNA nucleotide bases?

   a. rRNA

   b. mRNA

   c. tRNA

   d. nRNA

3. Your friend Shana is pregnant and wondering if there is anything she can do to increase her chances of having a girl. You tell her that the sex of the infant is determined:

   a. After transcription

   b. After translation

   c. By autosomes

   d. By sex chromosomes

4. An example of a trait that is affected by multifactorial inheritance would be:

   a. Eye color

   b. Hair color

   c. Blood type

   d. Height

5. When a nucleotide substitution occurs, this is called a(n):

   a. Genetic mutation

   b. Balanced translocation

   c. Epigenetic modification

   d. Nondisjuncture

6. Fay and Dan have recently visited a genetic counselor. The counselor told them that they were both carriers for an autosomal recessive genetic disorder. What are the chances that their child could express the disease?

   a. 0%

   b. 25%

   c. 50%

   d. 100%

7. In order for an individual to be considered as a carrier, they must be:

   a. Heterozygous for an autosomal dominant gene mutation

   b. Homozygous for an autosomal dominant gene mutation

   c. Homozygous for an autosomal recessive gene mutation

   d. Heterozygous for an autosomal recessive gene mutation

8. Which of the following nucleotide bases is found only in RNA?

   a. Adenine

   b. Thymine

   c. Uracil

   d. Guanine

9. Huntington disease is an example of a(n):

   a. Mitochondrial gene disorder

   b. Autosomal recessive disorder

   c. Autosomal dominant disorder

   d. Multifactorial recessive disorder

10. Folic acid is used for which of the following?

   a. Treatment of neural tube defects

   b. Prevention of neural tube defects

   c. Repair of DNA

   d. Correction of nondisjuncture

11. The chromosomal alteration that occurs with Down syndrome is:

    a. Imprinting of chromosome 21

    b. Balanced translocation of one copy of the chromosome 21

    c. One copy of chromosome 21

    d. Three copies of chromosome 21

12. Klinefelter syndrome is an example of a(n):

    a. Autosomal recessive disorder

    b. Autosomal dominant disorder

    c. Sex-linked disorder

    d. Carrier disorder

13. Which of the following is a manifestation of Turner syndrome?

    a. Amenorrhea

    b. Gynecomastia

    c. Tall stature

    d. Testicular atrophy

14. Cardiovascular disease is an example of a(n):

    a. Autosomal dominant genetic disorder

    b. Autosomal recessive genetic disorder

    c. Trisomy disorder

    d. Multifactorial disorder

15. Which of the following disorders is not hereditary?

    a. Sickle cell disease

    b. Fetal alcohol syndrome

    c. Fragile X syndrome

    d. Cystic fibrosis

Case Study 6.1

Ashland is a 24-year-old African American male with a history of sickle cell disease. Both of his parents have the sickle cell trait. Ashland has one brother who is not affected by sickle cell disease. Ashland has been admitted to the hospital numerous times over the past year due to sickle cell crisis. Ashland often has pain in his legs, back, and arms. He also suffers from fatigue related to anemia and he has frequent infections. Ashland is married and would like to have a large family.

1. *What is the type of alteration occurring within the body due to the genetic alteration in sickle cell disease? Describe the structure of the hemoglobin.*

2. *Discuss the occurrence and hereditary patterns of sickle cell disease.*

3. *Describe the cellular findings and clinical manifestations that Ashland is experiencing due to the sickle cell anemia. Draw a concept map of the alterations that are occurring within Ashland's body because of the sickle cell disease.*

4. *Discuss the treatments available for Ashland.*

Case Study 6.2

Lee is a 52-year-old male who has recently been diagnosed with Huntington disease. Lee is married and has 5 children. Some of his children have married and have children of their own. Lee is having muscle weakness and will often drop things he is holding. He is also having difficulty walking long distances. It is becoming difficult for Lee's wife to care for him at home due to his personality changes and loss of memory. She is afraid that he will wander away at night.

1. *What is the type of alteration occurring within the body due to the genetic alteration in Huntington disease?*

2. *Describe the mechanisms of dysfunction in this disorder. Draw a concept map linking the dysfunction to clinical manifestation.*

3. *Describe how Lee's children may benefit from genetic counseling. Would you recommend genetic testing for Lee's children and grandchildren? Why or why not?*

Concept Map Exercise

Drawing on what you have learned and studied in Chapter 6, fill in the missing terms in the concept map below.

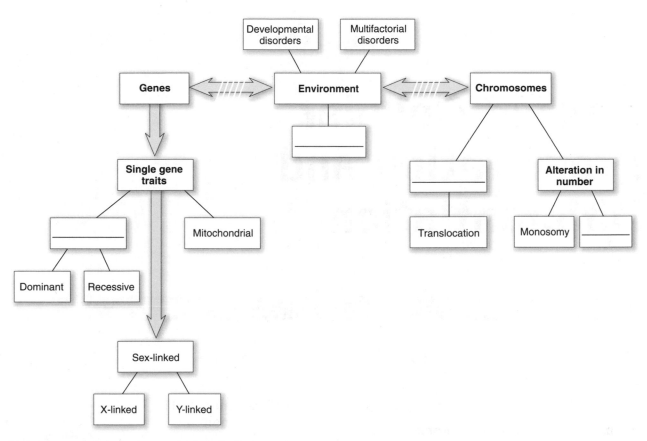

■ Concept map. Genetic alterations in human disease.

Altered Cellular Proliferation and Differentiation

KEY TERMS

adenocarcinoma

adenomas

anaplasia

autonomy

benign

blast cells

cachexia

cancer

carcinogen

carcinogenesis

carcinoma in situ

chondromas

chondrosarcoma

colonoscopy

crypts

differentiation

direct extension

ectopic

epistaxis

epithelioma

frank

grading

Hodgkin lymphoma

initiating event

local spread

malignant

metastases

monoclonal origin

mutator genes

neoplasms

non-Hodgkin lymphoma

occult

oncogenes

osteomas

palliative

papilloma

paraneoplastic
   syndromes

Philadelphia
   chromosome

progression

proliferation

promoting event

protooncogenes

Reed–Sternberg cell

seeding

staging

stem cells

teratomas

tropism

tumor markers

tumor suppressor genes

Chapter Review

1. Stem cells assist in the replacement of cells that have undergone necrosis or apoptosis. When the homeostasis of cell division is disrupted and there is a loss of regulated cell division, this results in:

   a. The overproliferation of cells

   b. Apoptosis

   c. Necrosis

   d. Differentiation

2. As cells grow and mature, they will typically develop specific characteristics and function. This type of orderly growth process is called:

   a. Proliferation

   b. Differentiation

   c. Adaptability

   d. Neoplasia

3. A type of cell that is highly undifferentiated that has the ability to mature into a differentiated cell with a specific function is called a:

   a. Transition cell

   b. Progenitor cell

   c. Stem cell

   d. Proliferation cell

4. When dividing cells have problems with overproliferation and lack of differentiation, this is called:

   a. Epithelial regression

   b. Mucosal irritation

   c. Neoplasia

   d. Stromal deviation

5. Tyrone, a 5-year-old has been diagnosed with a tumor in his brain. His parents are wondering what causes a tumor to form. You tell them that neoplastic growths occur when:

   a. There is hypoproliferation of cells

   b. There is epithelial regression

    c. Daughter cells are highly differentiated

    d. There is a loss of the regulatory mechanisms that rule cell behavior

6. We know that genetic mutations can play a role in the development of cancer. The three major categories of genes that can lead to cancerous transformations include all of the following except:

    a. Oncogenes

    b. Tumor suppressor genes

    c. Mutator genes

    d. Proliferation genes

7. Tumor suppressor genes play an active role in stopping overproliferation. The way that tumor suppressor genes manage potential overproliferation is through:

    a. Apoptosis

    b. Necrosis

    c. Cellular regression

    d. Proliferation stasis

8. Tyrone developed lung cancer from exposure to asbestos. Even after he was no longer exposed to the asbestos, the tumor continued to grow. When Tyrone's tumor no longer requires continued exposure to the cancer promoter (asbestos), this is called:

    a. Promotion

    b. Progression

    c. Proliferation

    d. Cell engagement

9. The long-term asbestos exposure ultimately affected Tyrone's lung tissue by causing long-term irritation. In response to this irritation, the cells attempted to adapt (metaplasia and dysplasia). An example of a cancer promoter that causes cellular changes over time is called:

    a. Cellular necrosis

    b. Inflammation

    c. Hyperpromotion

    d. Oncoproliferation

10. Genetics play a role in the development of cancer. Often, a single mutated cell is the origin of the cancer. This process where the cancer begins from a single mutated cell is called:

    a. Spontaneous mutation

    b. Proliferation transformation

    c. Mutation neoplasia

    d. Monoclonal origin

11. Cancer-causing agents such as radiation are called:

    a. Carcinogens

    b. Antigens

    c. Neoproliferators

    d. Oncogenetics

12. Neoplastic cells cause damage to normal tissue in many ways including all of the following except:

    a. Deprive unaffected tissues of oxygen

    b. Secrete substances that can alter metabolic processes

    c. Deprive healthy cells of nutrients

    d. Hypercellular communication

13. Tyrone's tumor in his lung was identified as malignant. Characteristics that are used to classify a tumor as malignant include all of the following except:

    a. Invasive

    b. Destructive

    c. High degree of differentiation

    d. No resemblance to the tissue of origin

14. After many rounds of chemotherapy and radiation therapy, it was determined that Tyrone's tumor was no longer treatable. When the treatment or care for cancer is primarily concerned with managing symptoms, this is called:

    a. Urgent care

    b. Palliative care

    c. Nonemergent care

    d. Preventive care

15. The main difference between childhood cancers and adult cancers is:

    a. Childhood cancers originate in the mesodermal germ layer

    b. Childhood cancers are metastatic in nature

    c. Adult cancers are slower growing

    d. Adult cancers initiate cellular differentiation

Case Study 7.1

Corrine is a 50-year-old female. She has made an appointment with her health care provider for a physical because of a recent, unintentional weight loss. During her appointment, Corrine tells her provider that she has had a change in her bowel habits over the past 6 months. She has also noted red blood in her bowel movements occasionally. Corrine also expresses the fact that she often has abdominal discomfort and feels very tired. Corrine tells her provider that she is worried about colon cancer because she has two brothers who have been diagnosed with colorectal cancer. Corrine was scheduled for a colonoscopy. During the colonoscopy a biopsy was taken from a growth identified in the colon. The pathology report identified cancer cells.

1. Compare a healthy cell in the lining of the colon to a cancerous one. What types of cellular changes take place in a malignant cell?

2. Draw a picture of a malignant cell in the colon. As you do this, consider the following: As the cancerous cells proliferate, how will the tumor affect the body locally (within the colon) and systemically?

3. Consider the location of the cancer and the surrounding structures. Where are the most likely sites of metastasis for Corrine? Why?

4. List the treatments available for Corrine and comment briefly on their potential effectiveness.

5. What risk factors for colon cancer does Corrine have?

Case Study 7.2

Irene is a 55-year-old female who has not been seen by a health care provider for the past 3 years. Irene lives an active lifestyle. She tries to eat a healthy diet and exercise. Irene plays tennis three times a week with her friends and tries to go for a short walk every day. Irene is being seen in the clinic today for her cough. Irene tells the health care provider that she had a "cold" 2 months ago and just cannot seem to get rid of the cough. Irene also reports feeling more fatigued and short of breath after playing tennis with her friends. Irene also reports chest pain when she takes a deep breath. The health care provider orders a chest X-ray and notes a rather large mass in the right lung. Arrangements are made for a biopsy of the mass and the pathology report indicates that the mass is cancerous.

1. Draw a concept map of the alteration that is occurring in Irene's body.

2. What types of clinical manifestations is Irene experiencing? Link those alterations to the clinical manifestations on your concept map.

3. Describe the relationship between the alteration and the clinical manifestations.

4. Describe the potential treatment options and discuss the rationale behind each treatment.

Concept Map Exercise

Drawing on what you have learned and studied in Chapter 7, fill in the missing terms in the concept map below.

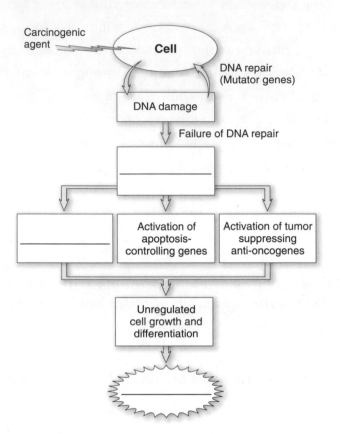

■ The genomic mechanisms of cancer. (Image modified from Porth CM. *Essentials of Pathophysiology: Concepts of Altered Health States*. Philadelphia: Lippincott Williams & Wilkins; 2003, with permission.)

Chapter 8

Altered Fluid, Electrolyte, and Acid–Base Balance

acid

amphoteric

anion exchange

anion gap

anions

anuria

aquaporins

ascites

bases

base deficit

base excess

buffer system

cations

cation exchange

cirrhosis

diuretics

electrolytes

extracellular compartment

filtration pressure

hepatic steatosis

hepatomegaly

hepatorenal syndrome

hydrostatic forces

hypercalcemia

hyperchloremia

hyperkalemia

hyperlactatemia

hypermagnesemia

hypernatremia

hyperphosphatemia

hypertonic

hypervolemia

hypocalcemia

hypochloremia

hypokalemia

hypomagnesemia

hyponatremia

hypophosphatemia

hypotonic

hypovolemia

intracellular compartment

ions

isotonic

lactic acidemia

lactic acidosis

loop diuretics

lymphedema

metabolic acidosis

metabolic alkalosis

nonvolatile acid	osmosis	portal hypertension
oliguria	osmotic pressure	Ringer's lactate
osmole	pH	thiazide diuretic
osmolality	paracentesis	turgor
osmolarity	parasthesia	urine specific gravity
osmoreceptors	pitting edema	volatile

Chapter Review

1. Two thirds of the body's total water is located in the:

   a. Intracellular compartment

   b. Extracellular compartment

   c. Vascular compartment

   d. Endothelial compartment

2. Ethel, your 80-year-old neighbor, just returned from a clinic visit. She tells you that she had her electrolytes drawn for a blood test. Ethel asks you what "electrolytes" are. You tell her that they are:

   a. Hypotonic particles

   b. Osmoreceptor particles

   c. Aquaporins

   d. Electrically charged particles known as ions

3. Antidiuretic hormone (ADH) helps maintain appropriate fluid levels in the body. ADH is released when there is a(n):

   a. Decreased blood osmolality

   b. Increased blood osmolality

   c. Ion gap

   d. Osmoreceptor decrease

4. Evelyn has increased fluid retention related to her congestive heart failure. Her health care provider would like to increase Evelyn's fluid excretion. The most common method for increasing fluid excretion includes the use of:

   a. Angiotensin

   b. Aldosterone

   c. Diuretics

   d. Aquaporins

5. Solutions that have a greater osmolality than the intracellular fluid (ICF) are called:

   a. Hypertonic

   b. Hypotonic

   c. Hyperactive

   d. Isotonic

6. Anne is experiencing a disruption in her pH balance. Which buffer system is the first to respond?

   a. Renal

   b. Plasma

   c. Respiratory

   d. Alkaline

7. The processes by which the kidneys contribute acids in order to maintain the pH balance include all of the following except:

   a. Secretion of hydrogen ions

   b. Reabsorption of sodium

   c. Production of ammonium ions

   d. Amphoteric secretion

8. Within the protein buffer system, albumin and plasma globulins can function as either acid or base. The term that describes this ability is:

   a. Amphoteric

   b. Nonvolatile

   c. Strong ion difference

   d. Osmotic absorption

9. The primary substances involved in the bicarbonate buffer system include:

   a. H_2CO_3

   b. $NaHCO_3$

   c. HCO_3

   d. a and b

   e. b and c

10. A potential problem that can occur as the potassium and hydrogen ion exchange attempts to maintain the pH balance is:

    a. Hypokalemia

    b. Hyperkalemia

    c. Hyponatremia

    d. Hypernatremia

11. Hypotonic hypovolemia is also known as:

    a. Edema

    b. Water detoxification

    c. Water intoxification

    d. Amphoteric intoxification

12. Hyponatremia causes cells to:

    a. Become hyperresponsive

    b. Remain static

    c. Swell

    d. Shrink

13. A mechanism contributing to the development of metabolic acidosis is:

    a. Decreased H^+ ions

    b. Increased HCO_3^- ions

    c. Loss of Cl^- ions

    d. Increase of Cl^- ions

14. In metabolic acidosis, there is a reduction of _____ and a(n) _____ in pH.

    a. HCO_3^-, increase

    b. Cl^-, decrease

    c. HCO_3^-, decrease

    d. $H_2CO_3^-$, decrease

15. In metabolic alkalosis, there is an increased level of _____ and a(n) _____ in the pH.

    a. HCO_3^-, decrease

    b. Cl^-, decrease

    c. HCO_3^-, increase

    d. $H_2CO_3^-$, decrease

Case Study 8.1

Lila is an 80-year-old female. Lila lives alone in her apartment. Over the weekend, Lila developed a cough and became increasingly short of breath. She also noticed that she had trouble putting her shoes on due to the swelling in her feet. Lila's daughter took her to the hospital where Lila was admitted for acute congestive heart failure.

1. *What are the active forces contributing to Lila's alteration in fluid balance associated with congestive heart failure?*

2. *What are the other manifestations that Lila may experience as a result of congestive heart failure–induced altered fluid balance?*

3. *What can be the treatment strategies used to restore Lila's fluid balance?*

4. *Consider the relationship between sodium and water. How is sodium especially critical to fluid balance?*

Concept Map Exercise

Drawing on what you have learned and studied in Chapter 8, fill in the missing terms in the concept map below.

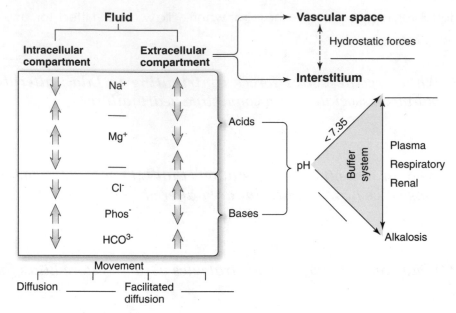

■ Fluid, electrolyte, and acid–base balance.

Chapter 9

Altered Neuronal Transmission

KEY TERMS

action potential

activities of daily living (ADLs)

affective disorder

afferent neurons

astrogliosis

ataxic

athetold

atrophy

autonomic nervous system (ANS)

autoreceptors

axon

axon hillock

blood–brain barrier (BBB)

blunt force injury

brachial plexus palsy

capacitor

cauda equina

cell body

central nervous system (CNS)

cerebral aqueduct

cerebrospinal fluid (CSF)

chemical synapse

choroid plexus

chromatolysis

clonic

closed head injury

communicating hydrocephalus

contralateral

corpus callosum

decerebrate posturing

decorticate posturing

demyelination

dendrites

depolarization

dermatomes

diplegia

distal axonopathy

dorsal horns

dyskinetic

efferent neurons

electrical synapses

encephalopathy

extrapyramidal disorders

extrapyramidal system

flaccid

functional electrical stimulation (FES)

ganglion

glia

global ischemia

glutamate

gray matter

gyri

hemiplegia

hyperpolarization

hypopolarization

interneuron

interventricular foramen

intraneuronal inclusions

lower motor neurons

membrane potential

meninges

microglial nodules

microstimulation

monoamines

mononeuropathy

motor neurons

N-methyl-D-aspartate
   (NMDA) receptor

neuromodulators

neuron

neuronophagia

neuronopathy

neuropathy

neurostimulation

neurotransmitters

nodes of Ranvier

noncommunicating
   hydrocephalus

nystagmus

oligodendrocytes

open traumatic injury

papilledema

parasympathetic
   nervous system (PNS)

paresthesia

peripheral nervous system

peripheral neuropathy

plexus

polyneuropathy

postictal

polarize

postganglionic neurons

preganglionic neurons

pseudobulbar affect

pyramidal motor system

quadriplegia

reflex arc

repolarization

resting membrane potential
   (RMP)

saltatory conduction

Schwann cells

sensory neurons

soma

somatic nervous system

spastic

subthreshold

sulci

sympathetic nervous system
   (SNS)

synapse

syndrome

threshold potential

thoracolumbar nervous

tonic

transillumination

upper motor neurons

ventral horns

ventricles

Wallerian degeneration

white matter

Chapter Review

1. Tom has difficulty moving and controlling his legs after a motor vehicle
   accident. The neurons most likely involved are called:

   a. Motor neurons

   b. Sensory neurons

   c. Afferent neurons

   d. Central neurons

2. The way that neurons communicate with other neurons and cells in the body is through:

   a. Subthresholds

   b. Schwann cells

   c. Oligodendrocytes

   d. Action potentials

3. The components of the action potential in the neuron include all of the following except:

   a. Resting membrane potential

   b. Depolarization phase

   c. Capacitor potential

   d. Repolarization phase

4. The small gap that separates neurons is called the:

   a. Neurotransmitter

   b. Synapse

   c. Dendrite

   d. Axon

5. Adrian suffered from a cerebral vascular accident (stroke). After the stroke, Adrian had difficulty with his reasoning ability and his speech. The part of his brain most likely affected by the stroke is:

   a. Frontal lobe

   b. Occipital lobe

   c. Parietal lobe

   d. Temporal lobe

6. Functions of the blood–brain barrier include all of the following methods of protection except:

   a. Protection of the brain from foreign substances

   b. Protection of the brain from hormones and neurotransmitters

   c. Protection against drastic environmental changes

   d. Protection from all bacteria

7. The cranial nerves mediate:

   a. Repolarization

   b. The glial response

   c. Sensory and motor functions

   d. Cerebral spinal fluid circulation

8. Cerebral spinal fluid is produced by the:

   a. Pia mater

   b. Choroid plexus

   c. Ventricles

   d. Meninges

9. Mary is experiencing a sympathetic response. You would expect to see all of the following except:

   a. Increased heart rate and contractility

   b. Smooth muscle relaxation of the bronchioles

   c. Vasoconstriction

   d. Constriction of the bronchiole smooth muscle

10. Anna has experienced damage to neurons in her brain due to Alzheimer disease. Her daughter asks you if Anna's body will ever be able to repair the damaged neurons. You know that:

    a. Mature neurons do not divide

    b. Sympathetic neurons divide

    c. Neurons are able to divide

    d. Only neurons in the afferent system can divide

11. Mark was in a motor vehicle accident and sustained a closed head injury. He hit his head on the steering wheel when his car hit a tree. The area where the initial impact occurred is called the:

    a. Contercoup

    b. Recoup

    c. Postcoup

    d. Coup

12. Cerebral palsy involves damage to the:

    a. Lower motor neurons

    b. Peripheral nervous system

    c. Upper motor neurons

    d. Motor neuron synapse

13. Rowan has multiple sclerosis. The symptoms that she is experiencing include cognitive loss, bowel and bladder dysfunction, altered mobility, and spasticity. The symptoms that Rowan is experiencing result from:

    a. Neuron tangles

    b. Synapse hyperreactivity

  c. Impairment in neurologic transduction

  d. Transmitter depolarization

14. Depression is recognized by a cluster of symptoms such as mood features and cognitive features. This cluster of symptoms is known as a:

  a. Symptom

  b. Clinical manifestation

  c. Sign

  d. Syndrome

15. Hydrocephalus is caused by:

  a. Communication of spinal fluid between the ventricles

  b. Increased cerebral spinal fluid excretion

  c. The accumulation of cerebral spinal fluid

  d. Increased cerebral spinal fluid absorption

Case Study 9.1

Marilyn is an active 49-year-old. Marilyn lives a very active lifestyle and enjoys swimming and biking. She works full time as an accountant and also volunteers when she can at the local food shelf. Lately, Marilyn has been having difficulty seeing the computer screen because of blurred vision. Marilyn has also noticed that she has been tripping quite frequently. In fact, last week when she was walking the dog, she tripped on the grass and injured her knee. It is becoming difficult for Marilyn to maintain her full load at work because she is so tired. Marilyn is being seen at the clinic today. Marilyn's health care provider suspects multiple sclerosis.

1. What alteration is occurring in Marilyn's body?

2. Draw a concept map of the neuronal alteration. How is the neuronal transmission pattern altered due to the multiple sclerosis?

3. Consider the clinical manifestations that Marilyn exhibits. Add these to your concept map and connect them with the alteration.

4. Is the alteration progressive or static? Describe the pattern.

5. Look at your concept map. What types of treatment might be implemented for Marilyn? What is the target for the treatment? What is the overall goal of the treatment for Marilyn?

Case Study 9.2

Shawnee and Tyrone have a 4-month-old baby boy, Ray. Ray was born with hydrocephalus. Since his birth, Ray has required increased visits to his pediatrician as well as surgery to place a shunt. At Ray's last visit, his length and weight were both in the 10th percentile on the growth chart. This means that Ray is normal, but smaller than most of the babies his age.

1. List the potential causes of hydrocephalus in an individual. Which of these is most likely the cause of Ray's hydrocephalus?

2. What type of alteration is occurring in hydrocephalus? Draw a concept map of the alteration.

3. What impact does the increased amount of cerebral spinal fluid have on the surrounding tissues? Add this to your concept map.

4. What clinical manifestations would Ray exhibit as the pressure increases in his brain?

5. Why did Ray's pediatrician utilize the placement of a shunt? Discuss the concerns and complications that may occur with a shunt.

▨ Concept Map Exercise

Drawing on what you have learned and studied in Chapter 9, fill in the missing terms in the concept map below.

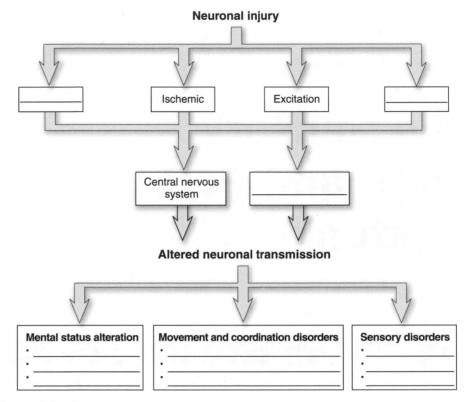

■ Mechanisms of neuronal disorders.

Chapter 10

Altered Sensory Function and Pain Perception

KEY TERMS

accommodate

acoustic reflex measurement

acuity

amblyopia

anterolateral pathway

aqueous humor

astigmatism

atrophic macular degeneration

barotrauma

body-self neuromatrix

cataracts

central auditory processing disorder

cerumen

choroidal neovascularization

ciliary body

ciliary muscles

cochlea

cochlear implants

conductive hearing loss

cones

conjunctivitis

cornea

decibels (dB)

diplopia

discriminative pathway

drusen

dry (atrophic) MD

electronystagmography (ENG)

endolymph

esotropia

external auditory meatus

fovea

gate control theory

glycerol test

Hertz (Hz)

hyperopia

incus

iris

irrigation

labrynthitis

lacrimal glands

laser-assisted in situ keratomileusis(LASIK)

lens

macula

malleus

mastoiditis

Ménière disease

mixed hearing loss

myofacia	oval window	specificity theory
myopia	pattern theory	stapes
neurogenic	pinna	strabismus
neuromatrix theory	presbycusis	substantia gelatinosa
neuropathic	presbyopia	thermoreceptor
nociceptive	pupil	tinnitus
nystagmus	pure tone bone conduction	trabecular network
olfaction		two-point discrimination
Organ of Corti	retina	tympanic membrane
ossicles	rhodopsin	tympanometry
otitis externa	rods	uveal-scleral outflow pathway
otitis media	sensorineural hearing loss	visual processing
otoacoustic emission (OAE)	somatosensory modalities	wet (exudative) MD
otosclerosis		

Chapter Review

1. Sensory receptors that are located in the skin and sense touch, pain, heat, and cold are called:

   a. Mechanoreceptors

   b. Chemoreceptors

   c. Osmoreceptors

   d. Photoreceptors

2. Neurons function in an orderly manner to relay information to the brain. Neurons that communicate sensory information from the periphery to the CNS are called:

   a. Second-order neurons

   b. First-order neurons

   c. Somatosensory neurons

   d. Mechanoreceptors

3. The pathway that communicates sensory information, including discriminative touch and spatial orientation, is called the:

   a. Second-order neuron pathway

   b. Dermatome pathway

   c. Sensory motor cortex pathway

   d. Discriminative pathway

4. All of the following are autonomic responses except:

   a. Dilation of pupils

   b. Constriction of blood vessels

   c. Dilation of blood vessels

   d. Increased heart rate

5. The somatosensory association areas in the nervous system assist with:

   a. The interpretation of stimuli into perceptions

   b. Blocking the discriminative pathway

   c. The dermatome system

   d. Triggering the autonomic nervous system

6. The area in the eye that is responsible for central vision, color vision, and fine detail is called the:

   a. Cornea

   b. Vitreous humor

   c. Pupil

   d. Macula

7. The extraocular muscles that control eye movement are innervated by:

   a. Dermatomes

   b. Macula ganglion

   c. Cranial nerves

   d. Ruffini's endings

8. Carrie's younger brother poked her in the right eye with his finger. Carrie runs to her mother. Carrie's mother observed an increased amount of tears in the right eye and wonders if this is normal. You tell her that the tears will help protect Carrie's eye in all of the following ways except:

   a. Protecting against bacterial infection

   b. Providing nutrients and moisture

   c. Increasing extraocular pressure

   d. Removing debris and waste from the eye

9. The aqueous humor performs the following function within the eye:

   a. Assists with lubrication of the sclera

   b. Provides protection from bacterial infection

   c. Triggers the production of tears with injury to the eye

   d. Maintains eye pressure and provides nutrients to the cornea

10. Anthony's teacher called his mother and stated that he was having difficulty seeing things on the whiteboard at school. After seeing an optometrist, Anthony was diagnosed with myopia. This type of error in vision is called a(n):

    a. Refraction error

    b. Strabismus error

    c. Oculomotor error

    d. Cranial nerve disruption error

11. Anthony also has an alteration within his eye that affects the coordination of the extraocular muscles resulting in double vision. This is called:

    a. Astigmatism

    b. Diplopia

    c. Oculopia

    d. Strabismus

12. As Tom's health care provider is checking the coordination of his eye movements, she notices involuntary oscillations of the eye. These involuntary oscillations are called:

    a. Conjunctivitis

    b. Amblyopia

    c. Nystagmus

    d. Esotropia

13. Katelynn's mother brings her in to see her health care provider. Upon examination, the provider observes that the sclera of Katelynn's left eye is reddened with excessive watering. There is no redness observed in her right eye. Katelynn denies the sensation of itching in her eyes. The type of conjunctivitis that Katelynn has is most likely:

    a. Bacterial

    b. Viral

    c. Allergic

    d. Inflammatory

14. Cataracts cause alteration in vision in the following way:

   a. They scatter the incoming light onto the retina

   b. They allow increased amounts of light into the pupil

   c. They obstruct the extraocular muscles

   d. They damage the retina through increased intraocular pressure

15. When Anthony saw his optometrist, she evaluated his visual acuity. This examination was most likely accomplished through:

   a. Observation of the pupil reaction

   b. Examination of the retina

   c. Dilation of the pupil

   d. The use of a Snellen chart

Case Study 10.1

Shane is a happy 6-month-old baby. He has had a cold for the past week. Amanda, his mother, brought him into urgent care this evening stating that he had a fever when she picked him up from daycare this afternoon. She also states that Shane does not want to nurse and that he has been crying most of the afternoon. Shane has been very healthy and aside from a few colds, he hasn't had any other problems. Upon examination, the health care provider noted that Shane's right tympanic membrane was red and bulging. Shane was diagnosed with acute otitis media.

1. Describe the alteration occurring within Shane's ear. How will this alteration affect Shane's sensation of hearing?

2. Discuss the manifestations that Shane is experiencing related to the acute otitis media.

3. Explore the treatment options for acute otitis media.

4. Consider the effects of repeated otitis media. What alterations will occur in relation to the repeated inflammation of the tympanic membrane?

Case Study 10.2

Ruby is a 70-year-old female. Ruby enjoys visiting her grandchildren. Ruby also enjoys traveling and she is worried about her ability to drive as she has noticed some "blind" spots in the periphery of her visual fields. She denies any pain. Ruby has a history of diabetes, hypertension, and obesity. Ruby has scheduled a routine visit to see her ophthalmologist. Her ophthalmologist has diagnosed her with primary open angle glaucoma.

1. *Describe the pathophysiologic process that leads to glaucoma.*

2. *What risk factors does Ruby have that increase the likelihood of the development of glaucoma?*

3. *Consider the pathophysiology of glaucoma. Describe how the increased pressure within the eye damages adjacent cells and tissue.*

4. *Draw a concept map of the alteration that causes glaucoma. What clinical manifestations would you expect to see with this alteration? Connect these manifestations with the alteration.*

5. *Consider the concept map that you have drawn. What types of treatment could be considered for Ruby's glaucoma? How do these interventions target the alteration?*

Concept Map Exercise

Drawing on what you have learned and studied in Chapter 10, fill in the missing terms in the concept map below.

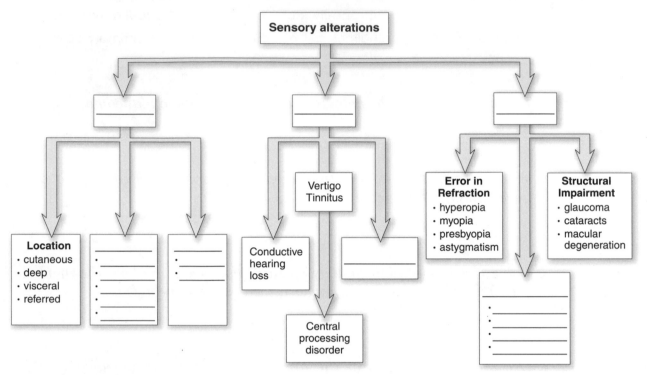

■ Sensory alterations.

Chapter 11

Altered Hormonal and Metabolic Regulation

KEY TERMS

acromegaly

Addison disease

cretinism

Cushing disease

Cushing syndrome

diabetes insipidus (DI)

endocrine system

exophthalmos

general adaptation
    syndrome

goiter

Grave disease

hirsutism

hormones

hyperpituitarism

hyperthyroidism

hypopituitarism

hypothalamic–pituitary
    axis

intertility

myxedema

negative feedback loop

panhypopituitarism

polyuria

positive feedback loop

stress

syndrome of
    inappropriate
    antidiuretic hormone
    (SIADH)

thyrotoxic crisis

thyrotoxicosis

Chapter Review

1. The initiation of hormone secretion and the regulation for hormones relies upon neuronal control through the:

   a. Anterior pituitary

   b. Posterior pituitary

   c. Hypothalamic-pituitary axis

   d. Paracrine pathways

2. The primary mechanism for the regulation of hormone levels in the blood is referred to as the:

   a. Negative feedback loop

   b. Positive feedback loop

   c. Environmental feedback loop

   d. Pituitary axis feedback loop

3. The process that allows hormones to act upon some cells and not others is called:

   a. Positive feedback

   b. Protein binding

   c. Pituitary axis feedback binding

   d. Receptor binding

4. The stress response is coordinated by the:

   a. Central nervous system

   b. Neuroendocrine system

   c. Endocrine pathway

   d. Autocrine pathway

5. The neuroendocrine response to a stressor and the physiologic changes that occur as a result of the stressor is called the:

   a. Alarm syndrome

   b. Positive feedback loop

   c. General adaptation syndrome

   d. Negative feedback loop

6. Periods of persistent stress are generally followed by the resistance stage. This stage is characterized by:

   a. Decreased levels of cortisol

   b. Increased levels of cortisol

   c. Increased receptor binding

   d. A decrease in the negative feedback loop

7. Aaron was out walking alone in the dark. When he heard a noise in the grass, Aaron's heart rate and respirations increased as his body prepared to defend itself. This stage in the general adaptation syndrome is called the:

   a. Alarm stage

   b. Resistance stage

   c. Preparation stage

   d. Flight stage

8. Hormone deficits and loss of hormone stimulation are the result of disturbance in:

   a. Hyperthalamic function

   b. Hypothalamic function

   c. The general adaptation syndrome

   d. The limbic system

9. Rose has a deficiency of all anterior pituitary hormones. This type of deficiency is called:

   a. Hyperpituitarism

   b. Hypopituitarism

   c. Panhypopituitarism

   d. Pituitary deficit

10. In the syndrome of inappropriate antidiuretic hormone (SIADH), there is:

    a. Excessive production and release of antidiuretic hormone

    b. Hyposecretion of antidiuretic hormone

    c. Decreased absorption of antidiuretic hormone

    d. Increased release of thyrotropin

11. Carol has the condition known as diabetes insipidus. She has a large volume of urine output. The loss of fluids and subsequent dehydration leads to:

    a. Serum hyperosmolality

    b. Serum hypoosmolality

    c. Concentrated urine

    d. High specific gravity of urine

12. The release of thyroid hormones from the thyroid gland is triggered by:

    a. Thyrocytes

    b. Thyrotoxicosis

    c. Glucocorticoids

    d. Thyroid-stimulating hormone

13. Andrew has been diagnosed with Cushing syndrome. In this condition, there is an excess secretion of:

    a. Glucocorticoids

    b. Androgens

    c. Aldosterone

    d. Epinephrine

14. Roland has exophthalmos. He also experienced weight loss, agitation, and restlessness. All of these manifestations are characteristic of:

    a. SIADH

    b. Diabetes insipidus

    c. Hypothyroidism

    d. Graves disease

15. The antidiuretic hormone helps to promote water retention by:

    a. Decreasing sodium retention

    b. Increasing the permeability of the nephrons in the kidneys

    c. Decreasing perfusion to the kidneys

    d. Decreasing blood pressure

Case Study 11.1

Donna is a 35-year-old construction worker. She has noted a 20-pound weight loss over the past 3 months. Donna also complains of being restless and unable to tolerate the heat when she is out on the construction site. Donna's menstrual cycle has become irregular and she wonders if she is beginning menopause. Upon examination, Donna's thyroid gland was enlarged. Lab tests confirmed the diagnosis of Graves disease.

1. *Discuss the alteration within the endocrine system that occurs with Graves disease.*

2. *What are the potential reasons for altered hormonal regulation for Donna?*

3. *Discuss the immunologic mechanism that is a catalyst for Graves disease.*

4. *Consider the clinical manifestations that Donna is experiencing. How does the altered hormonal and metabolic regulation impact Donna's normal body processes?*

5. *What diagnostic tests were most likely ordered to determine the diagnosis for Donna?*

Concept Map Exercise

Drawing on what you have learned and studied in Chapter 11, fill in the missing terms in the concept map below.

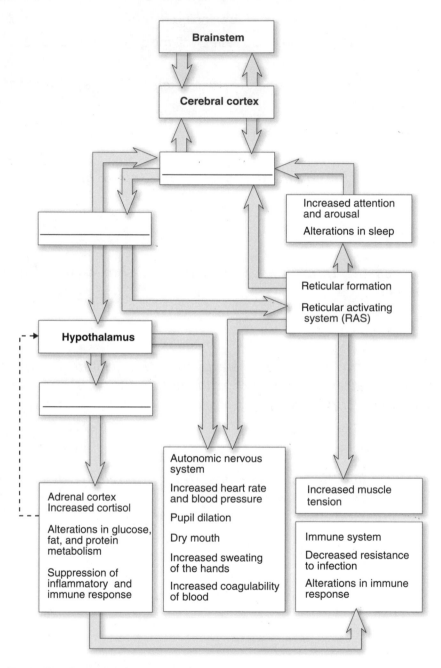

■ Stress pathways. The broken line represents negative feedback. (Image modified from Porth CM. *Essentials of Pathophysiology: Concepts of Altered Health States*. Philadelphia: Lippincott Williams and Wilkins; 2003, with permission.)

Chapter 12

Altered Reproductive Function

KEY TERMS

amenorrhea

anovulation

atretic

cryptorchidism

dysmenorrhea

dyspareunia

embryonic
  carcinomas

endometriosis

erectile
  dysfunction (ED)

leiomyomas

menarche

menopause

menorrhagia

metrorrhagia

metromenorrhagia

oligomenorrhea

perimenopause

polymenorrhea

polycystic ovary
  syndrome (PCOS)

spermatogonia

teratocarcinomas

Chapter Review

1. Your friend is concerned because she has not yet conceived. She tells you that she has been trying for the past 4 months without success and thinks that she is infertile. Which of the following is true about the definition of infertility?

   a. The inability to conceive after 12 months is descriptive of infertility

   b. Infertility is not defined by a timeline

   c. She probably has a fallopian tube obstruction since this is the most common cause

   d. None of these are true

2. Several months later, your friend again comes to you with the same concern of infertility. You recommend that they both go in for an evaluation since she has not yet been able to conceive. What should they expect as the first step in the evaluation of infertility?

   a. Monitoring for signs of ovulation

   b. Sperm analysis

   c. Complete history and physical examinations

   d. All of these

3. Your friend tells you that her physician has recommended a hystero-salpinogram. She has no idea what this means. How do you explain it to her?

   a. This is an MRI of the reproductive structures

   b. This is a CT scan of the reproductive structures

   c. This is an X-ray of the reproductive structures using a contrast dye

   d. This is a form of diagnostic laporoscopy where internal reproductive structures are visualized

4. Which of the following risk factors would increase the likelihood of infertility in females?

   a. Excessive exercise and low body fat percentage

   b. Poor dietary calcium intake

   c. Completely treated pelvic infections

   d. Weekly intercourse

5. Your friend with infertility is told that she has thick, impenetrable cervical mucous. What is used to overcome this problem?

   a. In vitro fertilization

   b. Artificial insemination

   c. Use of clomiphene citrate

   d. Douching

6. Which of the following is not likely to result in infertility?

   a. Spermatazoa aging

   b. The male partner has a varicocele

   c. Use of lubricants during intercourse

   d. Erectile dysfunction

7. Which is a common microorganism responsible for pelvic inflammatory disease?

   a. Herpes virus

   b. Hemophilus influenza type B

   c. Streptococcus

   d. Gonorrhea

8. Which of the following patients should be hospitalized if diagnosed with pelvic inflammatory disease?

   a. All patients with PID should be hospitalized

   b. Pregnant patient

   c. Teenage patient

   d. Patient with a temperature of 99.6 °F

9. What problem category of infertility would describe pelvic inflammatory disease?

   a. Obstructive

   b. Hormonal

   c. Invasive

   d. Motility

10. What problem category of infertility would describe polycystic ovarian syndrome?

   a. Obstructive

   b. Hormonal

   c. Invasive

   d. Motility

11. Which of the following does not occur with polycystic ovarian syndrome?

   a. Ovulation

   b. Hursuitism

   c. Multiple immature follicles

   d. Constant estrogen production

12. In PCOS, a relationship has been noted between high androgen levels and insulin resistance, where insulin excess promotes excessive _____.

   a. Pituitary secretion of LH

   b. Ovarian secretion of androgens

   c. Hypothalamis secretion of GnRH

   d. Ovarian secretion of FSH

13. What treatment is needed for women with PCOS?

   a. Ovarian dissection

   b. Artificial insemination

   c. Antiestrogen medications

   d. In vitro fertilization

14. Which of the following is the most common form of ovarian cancer?

   a. Adenocarcinoma

   b. Germ cell tumors

   c. Sex cord tumors

   d. Myeloma

15. Your neighbor tells you that she has stage IV ovarian cancer. What does this mean?

   a. The cancer is isolated to both ovaries

   b. There are distant metastases

   c. The tumor is benign

   d. The ovarian cancer has extended into the pelvis

16. The loss of the trophic stimulation of the hormones associated with ovarian cycles precipitates atrophic changes in the cells of the reproductive organs leading to _____.

    a. Menopause

    b. Menarche

    c. Dyspareunia

    d. Peritonitis

17. Which of the following is not a hormonal factor attributed to erectile dysfunction?

    a. Spinal cord injury

    b. Hypogonadism

    c. Hypothyroidism

    d. Adrenal cortical hormone dysfunction

18. How common is benign prostatic hypertrophy?

    a. Very rare; about 5% of men over 50

    b. Fairly common; about 50% of men over 70

    c. Very common; about 70% of men over 70

    d. Extremely common; about 90% of men over 70

19. Which men are appropriate candidates for treatment of BPH?

    a. All men should be treated

    b. Those with significant symptoms

    c. Those with elevated PSA levels

    d. Those with urinary frequency

Case Study 12.1

Joan is a 49-year-old married woman with four children. She works full time as an office manager in a small software company. During her routine yearly physical, you ask about her menstrual cycles. Joan tells you that she has noticed that they have become irregular with heavier bleeding at times. Her last menstrual period was 3 months ago. She also complains of vaginal dryness, fatigue, and mood swings. Joan asks you if she could possibly be entering menopause. She indicates concern about the changes her body is going through and wonders how this will affect her relationship with her husband. An FSH and estradiol blood levels were drawn.

1. What signs and symptoms are associated with menopause?

2. *What do you suspect Joan's FSH and estradiol blood levels will be? Why?*

3. *What is the alteration that is occurring in Joan's body? Why is this significant? How did Joan's body respond to this alteration?*

4. *Consider Joan's concern about how menopause will affect her relationship with her husband. How would you respond?*

5. *Create a concept map of the structural and functional changes taking place within Joan's body during menopause. Next, add Joan's signs and symptoms to the concept map. Connect the signs and symptoms with the structural and functional changes taking place.*

█ Concept Map Exercise

Drawing on what you have learned and studied about polycystic ovarian syndrome in Chapter 12, fill in the missing terms in the concept map below.

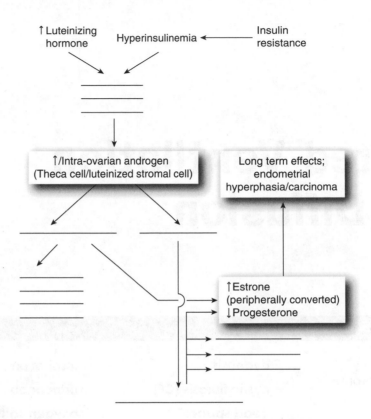

█ Pathogenesis of polycystic ovary syndrome. (Image from Rubin E, Farber JL. *Pathology*. 3rd ed. Philadelphia: Lippincott Williams & Wilkins; 1999, with permission.)

Chapter 13

Altered Ventilation and Diffusion

KEY TERMS

acute respiratory distress syndrome (ARDS)

adventitious

air trapping

anoxia

aspiration

asthma

atelectasis

atopic

auscultation

bronchiectasis

caseous necrosis

cavitation

chronic bronchitis

chronic obstructive pulmonary disease (COPD)

clubbing

compliance

consolidation

cyanosis

cystic fibrosis (CF)

dead space

diffusing capacity

diffusion

dyspnea

emphysema

expectorate

expiration

forced expiratory volume in 1 second (FEV_1)

forced vital capacity (FVC)

fully saturated

Ghon complex

Ghon focus

hemoptysis

hypercapnia

hypoxemia

hypoxia

inspiration

orthopnea

oxygen saturation (SaO_2)

oxyhemoglobin (HbO_2)

$PaCO_2$

PaO_2

partial pressure

perfusion

phlegm

pneumonia

pneumothorax

pursed lip breathing

residual volume (RV)

respiration

respiratory failure

retractions

sputum

status asthmaticus

surfactant

tidal volume (TV)   tuberculosis (TB)   vital capacity (VC)

total lung capacity (TLC)   ventilation

Chapter Review

1. Respiration differs from ventilation in that respiration involves:

   a. The movement and exchange of oxygen in the alveoli

   b. Supplying oxygenated blood to the lungs and organ systems

   c. The mechanical process of moving air in and out of the respiratory system

   d. All of the body's cells and the utilization of oxygen to make energy

2. Ethan is sitting next to Ryan in class. Ethan has a cold and is coughing. Ryan is worried about catching a cold. You tell Ryan that the pulmonary system has defense mechanisms to help him stay healthy. These defense mechanisms include all of the following except:

   a. Macrophages in the alveoli

   b. Chemoreceptors

   c. Structural protections such as hair

   d. Mucosal lining that has an immune coating

3. Todd is competing in a 2K run for his track team. As Todd is completing his laps on the track, his body is regulating the rate and volume of his respirations. All of the following are important in this regulation except:

   a. Lung receptors

   b. Respiratory control center in the brain

   c. Diffusing capacity

   d. Chemoreceptors

4. After surgery, Myron needed to have the oxygen saturation in his blood monitored for potential hypoxemia. The method most likely used in monitoring Myron is called:

   a. Pulse oximetry

   b. Ventilation oximetry

c. Respiration observation

d. Diffusion oximetry

5. When the body cannot maintain homeostasis because of an alteration in ventilation and diffusion, all of the following will occur except:

a. Hyperthermia

b. Hypercapnia

c. Hypoxia

d. Hypoxemia

6. Andrea is sitting quietly reading in her chair. The amount of air that Andrea exhales after passive inspiration is called:

a. Tidal volume

b. Vital capacity

c. Residual volume

d. Total lung capacity

7. The lipoprotein that coats the inner portion of the alveolus and promotes ease of expansion is called:

a. Ghon complex

b. Surfactant

c. Atopic protein

d. Marfan protein

8. Marlyn has pneumonia. He has decreased oxygen in the arterial blood and a decrease in the partial pressure of oxygen. This decreased oxygen level is called:

a. Hypoxia

b. Hypercapnea

c. Hypoxemia

d. Aspiration

9. Because of Marlyn's pneumonia and the increased collection of fluid/pus in the alveoli, he will most likely experience impaired:

a. Inspiration

b. Expiration

c. Ventilation

d. Diffusion

10. Marlyn is experiencing a deprivation of adequate oxygen to his cells. This is called:

    a. Hypoxia

    b. Hypercapnea

    c. Hypoxemia

    d. Aspiration

11. Marlyn is admitted to the hospital because of his pneumonia. He has impaired diffusion and ventilation with an increased amount of carbon dioxide level in his blood. This increased level of carbon dioxide in the blood is called:

    a. Hypoxia

    b. Hypercapnea

    c. Hypoxemia

    d. Aspiration

12. Marlyn experienced many local manifestations related to impaired ventilation and diffusion. All of the following would be considered local manifestations except:

    a. Fever

    b. Cough

    c. Dyspnea

    d. Excess mucous production

13. Marlyn complains of increased difficulty breathing when he is in a supine position and he prefers to have the head of his bed elevated. This need to sit upright is called:

    a. Dyspena

    b. Hypoxemia

    c. Hyperventilation

    d. Orthopnea

14. Anthony is experiencing an acute exacerbation of his asthma. When you observe his chest, you notice that he is using accessory muscles during respiration and observe a pulling in of his intercostal muscles. You would describe this as:

    a. Orthopnea

    b. Subtractions

    c. Retractions

    d. Interactions

15. When you auscultate Anthony's lung sounds, you hear wheezing. Altered breath sounds such as this are called:

   a. Cavitations

   b. Inspiration

   c. Adventitious

   d. Ventilation

Case Study 13.1

Marie is 77 years old. She has a history of asthma that is well controlled. Marie has just returned from a vacation with her grandchildren. Shortly after returning home from her vacation, Marie noticed a productive cough, fever, chills, fatigue, and tachypnea. During the night, Marie experienced orthopnea with increased shortness of breath. Marie decided to visit the urgent care center near her home. After the physical assessment, the health care provider ordered a number of tests, including a white blood cell count, chest X-ray, and sputum culture. Marie was diagnosed with left lower lobe pneumonia.

1. Describe the pathophysiologic process that is occurring within Marie's lungs.

2. Describe the potential etiology, risk factors, and expected course for Marie.

3. What body processes are affected by the pneumonia? How does the pneumonia impact those processes?

4. List the clinical manifestations that you would expect to see with pneumonia. Which ones are local? Systemic?

5. What are the possible options for treatment for Marie? Describe the expected outcomes or goals for treatment.

Concept Map Exercise

Drawing on what you have learned and studied in Chapter 13, fill in the missing terms in the concept map below.

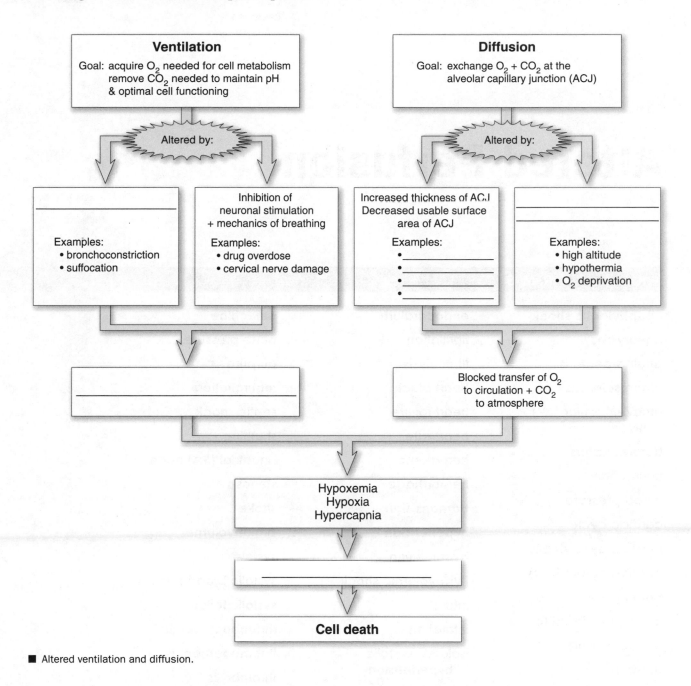

Ventilation
Goal: acquire O_2 needed for cell metabolism remove CO_2 needed to maintain pH & optimal cell functioning

Diffusion
Goal: exchange O_2 + CO_2 at the alveolar capillary junction (ACJ)

Altered by:

Altered by:

_____

Examples:
• bronchoconstriction
• suffocation

Inhibition of neuronal stimulation + mechanics of breathing

Examples:
• drug overdose
• cervical nerve damage

Increased thickness of ACJ Decreased usable surface area of ACJ

Examples:
• _____
• _____
• _____
• _____

_____

Examples:
• high altitude
• hypothermia
• O_2 deprivation

_____

Blocked transfer of O_2 to circulation + CO_2 to atmosphere

Hypoxemia
Hypoxia
Hypercapnia

_____

Cell death

■ Altered ventilation and diffusion.

Chapter 14

Altered Perfusion

KEY TERMS

anaphylactic shock

aneurysms

angina pectoris

atherosclerosis

atrioventricular (AV)
  node

baroreceptors

bifurcations

blood pressure

cardiac cycle

cardiac dysrhythmias

cardiac output (CO)

cardiogenic shock

congestive heart failure

cor pulmonale

diastole

diastolic blood pressure

diastolic failure

disseminated
  intravascular
  coagulation (DIC)

ecchymoses

embolus

endocardium

fibrillation

fibrinolysis

heart block

heart failure

heart rate

hematoma

hemorrhage

Homans sign

hypertension

hypotension

hypovolemic shock

infarct

infarction

isolated systolic
  hypertension

mean arterial pressure

myocardial infarction

myocardium

neurogenic shock

perfusion

pericardium

petechiae

pulse pressure

purpura

regurgitation

septic shock

shunting

sinoatrial (SA) node

stenosis

stroke

stroke volume

systole

systolic blood pressure

systolic failure

thrombocythemia

thromboembolus

thrombosis

transient ischemic
  attack (TIA)

ventilation–perfusion
  ratio

venous stasis

Virchow triad

Chapter Review

1. The lining of the heart that forms a first line of defense against infection and inflammation is called the:

   a. Exocardium

   b. Myocardium

   c. Endocardium

   d. Pericardium

2. A complete cardiac cycle includes:

   a. One contraction and one relaxation phase

   b. Two contractions and one relaxation phase

   c. One contraction and two relaxation phases

   d. Two contractions and two relaxation phases

3. The _____ of the heart contracts and relaxes.

   a. Myocardium

   b. Pericardium

   c. Endocardium

   d. Osteocardium

4. Jennifer tells you that she had to have an ECG yesterday. She asks what this test measures. You tell her that it measures:

   a. The myocardium thickness

   b. The resting phase of the myocardium

   c. The blood level in the heart

   d. The electrical activity of the heart

5. Match the following ECG characteristics to the source:

   _____ P Wave   _____ PQ interval

   _____ QRS   _____ T

   _____ U

   a. Depolarization of the AV node and bundle fibers

   b. Depolarization of the ventricles

    c. Repolarization of Purkinje fibers

    d. Depolarization of the atria via the SA node

    e. Repolarization of the ventricles

6. The following is considered the pacemaker of the heart:

    a. AV node

    b. BA node

    c. SA node

    d. Purkinje fibers

7. Raymond recently had a myocardial infarction and tells you that his cardiologist told him that his cardiac output is decreased. Raymond asks you what his cardiac output is. You tell him that it measures the:

    a. Heart's efficiency to pump optimal amounts of blood

    b. Number of heartbeats a minute

    c. Amount of blood that leaves the heart with each beat

    d. Pressure of the blood within the arteries

8. The systolic blood pressure measures:

    a. The difference between the diastolic and systolic pressure

    b. The amount of pressure that remains in the aorta during the resting phase of the cardiac cycle

    c. The amount of pressure exerted during contraction of the left ventricle

    d. The mean arterial pressure

9. These are located throughout the heart and they sense pressure changes in the arteries:

    a. Purkinje fibers

    b. RA node

    c. SA node

    d. Baroreceptors

10. The three major factors responsible for clot formation called Virchow triad include all of the following except:

    a. Vessel wall damage

    b. Excessive clotting

    c. Alterations in blood flow

    d. Hypocoagulation

11. Dale recently had a physical and was told by his physician's assistant that he had atherosclerosis. Dale is not sure what this means and asks you to explain it to him. You tell Dale that it is:

    a. Irregularly distributed lipid deposits in the inner lining of arteries

    b. An autoimmune mechanism

    c. A place where the vessel branches

    d. An outpouching in the vessel wall

12. David has had a myocardial infarction and has large infarct in the right atrium. An infarct is a(n):

    a. Area of necrosis due to an acute episode of insufficient blood supply

    b. Bifurcation of the artery

    c. Outpouching of the vessel wall

    d. Area of collateral circulation on the cardiac muscle

13. Blood movement across the chambers of the heart is referred to as:

    a. Shunting

    b. Regurgitation

    c. Stenosis

    d. Dysrhythmia

14. Elmer has a valve that is unable to close properly and allows reflux of blood. This is called:

    a. Shunting

    b. Regurgitation

    c. Stenosis

    d. Dysrhythmia

15. Carie has an allergy to penicillin. Her provider mistakenly prescribed this medication for her infection. Shortly after taking the medication, Carie experienced a massive immune hypersensitivity response and moved into a state of shock. This type of shock is called:

    a. Hypovolemic shock

    b. Septic shock

    c. Neurogenic shock

    d. Anaphylactic shock

Case Study 14.1

Meriam is an 80-year-old female. She has been independently living in her apartment. Meriam has a history of diabetes, hypertension, asthma, and obesity. Over the summer, Meriam noticed increased periods of shortness of breath with activity. She also noted a 10 pound weight gain over a 2-week period with a progressive cough. Meriam went to the clinic and had a series of tests ordered. Ultimately, Meriam was diagnosed with acute congestive heart failure and was hospitalized in order to manage the heart failure.

1. *What body processes are being affected by Meriam's heart failure? In what way does the heart failure impact those processes?*

2. *What clinical manifestations is Meriam experiencing? How are they related to the alteration that is occurring within her body?*

3. *What do you suspect is the etiology of Meriam's heart failure? Write a recipe for Meriam's heart failure.*

4. *Discuss the development of Meriam's heart failure. (Hint: Consider Meriam's risk factors.)*

5. *What types of care/support will Meriam most likely receive in the treatment of her heart failure?*

Case Study 14.2

Roman is a 70-year-old male. Roman has a history of hypertension and high cholesterol. Roman smokes one-half pack of cigarettes a day. He often doesn't take his antihypertensive medication because he doesn't think he needs it. Roman complained to his wife that he felt dizzy. Roman's wife also noted that his speech was slurred when he was talking to her and she noticed that the right side of his mouth was drooping. Roman's wife took him into urgent care. Roman was diagnosed with a stroke.

1. *What body processes are being altered by the stroke? In what way does the stroke impair those processes?*

2. *Describe how Roman's alteration in perfusion most likely developed. What are the important elements that must be present in order for a stroke to develop?*

3. *What clinical manifestations is Roman experiencing? How are the manifestations linked to the alteration in perfusion in the brain?*

4. *What part of Roman's brain is most likely experiencing the alteration in perfusion?*

5. *What types of tests might have been ordered to diagnose Roman's stroke? What treatments might be considered for Roman?*

Concept Map Exercise

Drawing on what you have learned and studied in Chapter 14, fill in the missing terms in the concept map below.

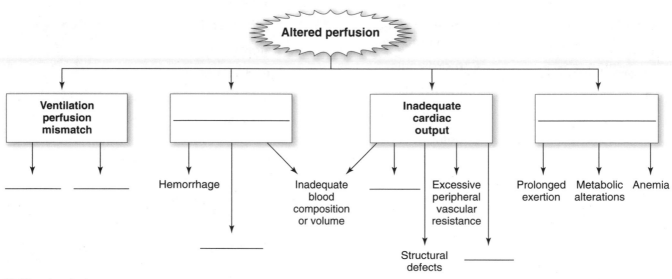

■ Altered perfusion.

Chapter 15

Altered Nutrition

KEY TERMS

active transport

absorption

anemia

anorexia nervosa

bioavailability

body mass index (BMI)

celiac disease

digestion

energy

essential nutrients

glutens

hypochromic

iron-deficiency anemia

kwashiorkor

lacteal

lanugo

lipids

macronutrients

malabsorption

malabsorption syndrome

marasmus

microcytic

micronutrients

nutrient

nutrition

obesity

overnutrition

passive diffusion

pica

poikilocytosis

satiety

saturated fatty acids

storage fat

undernutrition

unsaturated fatty acids

vitamins

Chapter Review

1. Examples of macronutrients include all of the following except:
   a. Proteins
   b. Carbohydrates
   c. Fats
   d. Vitamins

2. Fatty acids that elevate blood cholesterol are called:
   a. Saturated fatty acids
   b. Unsaturated fatty acids
   c. Monosaccharides
   d. Polysaccharides

3. The largest single component of the body is:
   a. Macronutrients
   b. Micronutrients
   c. Water
   d. Essential nutrients

4. When dietary carbohydrates are digested, they are converted to:
   a. Glucose
   b. Sucrose
   c. Adipose
   d. Coenzymes

5. Inorganic substances that are critical to the regulation of cellular processes are called:
   a. Proteins
   b. Minerals
   c. Vitamins
   d. Fatty acids

6. Hunger and satiety are regulated by the:
    a. Blood sugar levels
    b. Thalamus
    c. Hypothalamus
    d. Cerebral cortex

7. All of the following are essential functions of the digestive system except:
    a. Digesting and extracting macronutrients
    b. Absorbing nutrients
    c. Forming a barrier against microorganisms and foreign materials
    d. Storage of nutrients

8. The walls of the gastrointestinal tract contain the following layers:
    a. Inner mucosa
    b. Submucosa
    c. Muscularis and serosa
    d. a and b
    e. All of the above

9. The process of the body when it takes in nutrients and moves these into circulation in order to be used by cells is called:
    a. Absorption
    b. Digestion
    c. Reabsorption
    d. Bioavailablility

10. A state of inadequate or excessive exposure to nutrients is called:
    a. Malabsorption
    b. Resorption
    c. Malnutrition
    d. Undernutrition

11. The major energy source for body tissues is:
    a. Carbohydrates
    b. Minerals
    c. Vitamins
    d. Glucose

12. When dietary glucose is unavailable, the body will attempt to manufacture glucose. This is called:

    a. Glucolysis

    b. Gluconeogenesis

    c. Malabsorption

    d. Marasmus

13. All of the following affect hemoglobin levels except:

    a. Altitude

    b. Gender

    c. The retention of vitamin A

    d. Pregnancy

14. In anorexia nervosa, these levels increase due to the stress of malnutrition:

    a. Vitamin E

    b. Cortisol

    c. Glucose

    d. Antidiuretic hormone

15. Celiac disease is caused by a(n):

    a. Vitamin A reabsorption

    b. Excess cortisol

    c. T-cell–mediated hypersensitivity

    d. Excessive carbohydrates

Case Study 15.1

Connie is a 35-year-old female of Western European heritage. She works full time as a nurse and has four children. Over the past couple of years, Connie has noticed increased gastrointestinal symptoms of bloating, gas, and abdominal discomfort. Connie notices that the symptoms are more prevalent when she eats meals that contain a lot of carbohydrates. She is especially bothered when she eats bread or pasta. Connie was diagnosed with celiac disease.

1. Describe the alteration occurring within Connie's body. What body processes are affected?

2. *What is the most likely cause of Connie's celiac disease? How did it develop? What risk factors did Connie have?*

3. *What types of chronic complications occur with celiac disease? What complications is Connie experiencing?*

4. *What clinical manifestations would you expect to see with celiac disease?*

5. *How is celiac disease diagnosed? What test might have been ordered for Connie?*

Concept Map Exercise

Drawing on what you have learned and studied in Chapter 15, fill in the missing terms in the concept map below.

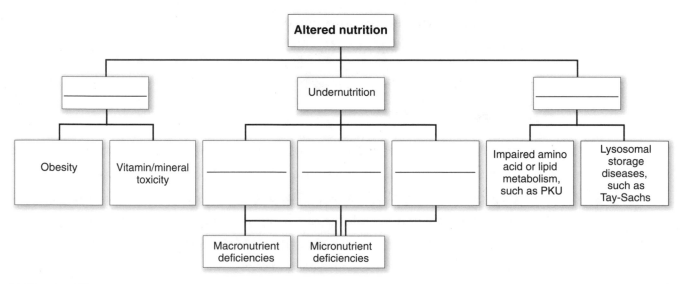

■ Altered nutrition.

Chapter 16

Altered Elimination

KEY TERMS

acute tubular necrosis

arteriovenous (AV) fistula

arteriovenous shunt

auscultation

bladder

bladder training

bowel resection

casts

colostomy

costovertebral angle (CVA)

countercurrent exchange

countercurrent mechanism

countercurrent multiplier

defecation

detrusor muscle

diverticula

diverticulitis

diverticulosis

diverticulum

encopresis

enteric nervous system

enuresis

external anal sphincter

external urethral sphincter

extracorporeal shockwave lithotripsy (ESWL)

functional incontinence

functional nonretentive soiling

glomerulus

haustras

hemodialysis

hydroureter

internal rectal sphincter

internal urethral sphincter

large intestine/colon

macroscopic analysis

mass movements

meconium

Meissner's plexus

melena

micturition

myenteric (Auerbach) plexus

nephron

occult

overactive bladder

overflow incontinence

paralytic ileus

percutaneous nephrolithotomy

peristalsis

peritoneal dialysis

peritonitis

polycystic kidney disease (PKD)

rectal reflex

retentive incontinence

segmental movement

steatorrhea

stercobilin

stress incontinence

struvite

teniae coli

trigone

urge incontinence

urine

urine dipstick

ureteroscopic stone
removal

Valsalva maneuvers

Chapter Review

1. The functional unit of the kidney is called the:

   a. Nephron

   b. Medulla

   c. Cortex

   d. Proximal tubule

2. In the kidney, reabsorption of water is accomplished with the help of:

   a. Renin

   b. Antidiuretic hormone

   c. Angiotensin

   d. Aldosterone

3. The smooth area at the base of the bladder between the openings of the two ureters and the urethra that serves as a functional sphincter is called:

   a. Internal sphincter

   b. Detrusor

   c. Trigone

   d. External sphincter

4. A newborn's first stool is called:

   a. Micturition

   b. Stercobilin

   c. Defecation

   d. Meconium

5. Accumulation of fluid in the urinary ureter is called:

   a. Hydronephrosis

   b. Tubular necrosis

c. Hydroureter

d. Reflux

6. Amy has a history of kidney disease. She is being seen at the clinic for oliguria. This means that Amy:

   a. Has scant urinary output

   b. Has no urine production

   c. Has reflux

   d. Has increased urinary output

7. Terri has a kidney infection. She complains of pain in the costovertebral area. This area is located in the:

   a. Right upper abdomen

   b. Umbilical area

   c. Flank area

   d. Right lower abdomen

8. Ruby has had a history of black stools (melena). This is indicative of:

   a. Renal colic

   b. Diarrhea

   c. Constipation

   d. The presence of blood in the stool

9. Andrew suffered from an intestinal perforation because of an obstruction. Because of the perforation, Andrew is at risk for developing:

   a. Steatorrhea

   b. Diarrhea

   c. Peritonitis

   d. Constipation

10. All of the following are chemical mediators of pain except:

    a. Progesterone

    b. Serotonin

    c. Bradykinin

    d. Histamine

11. Josh was seen by his provider for his routine physical. He was sent home with instructions to collect stool samples to check for occult blood in his stools. He asks you what occult blood is. You tell him that:

    a. It is bleeding from the lower GI tract

    b. It is traces of blood too small to be seen

    c. It is bleeding from the upper GI tract

    d. It is caused by constipation

12. Seth has constipation. His provider is treating him with bulk-forming laxatives. These work by:

    a. Increasing peristalsis

    b. Absorbing water into the intestine to make the stool softer

    c. Providing a stimulant effect

    d. Enhancing propulsion of the stool

13. Rita has diarrhea. A type of diet that is easily digested is called the:

    a. BRAT diet

    b. TOAST diet

    c. RICE diet

    d. LIQUID diet

14. Brad has severe right flank pain with nausea. He was diagnosed with urolithiasis. This means that he has:

    a. A bladder infection

    b. Kidney stones

    c. A kidney infection

    d. Reflux

15. Mary has had five children. She has problems with incontinence when she coughs or sneezes. What type of incontinence is this?

    a. Functional incontinence

    b. Overflow incontinence

    c. Urge incontinence

    d. Stress incontinence

Case Study 16.1

Tom is a 33-year-old man who went to the emergency department because of severe right flank pain. He is doubled over on the bed, writhing in pain. He is also experiencing nausea. Tom states that the pain woke him up from sleep and that he has never experienced the pain before. Tom is otherwise healthy and lives a very active lifestyle. He maintains a healthy diet. Tom drinks at least four glasses of milk a day, eats lots of beets (his favorite food), nuts and spinach, and takes calcium supplements. Tom is diagnosed with urolithiasis.

1. *Describe the alteration occurring within Tom's body. What body processes are affected?*

2. *What is the most likely cause of Tom's kidney stones? How did they develop? What risk factors did Tom have?*

3. *What types of chronic complications occur with kidney stones?*

4. *What clinical manifestations would you expect to see with kidney stones? Relate these to Question 1.*

5. *What are the current treatments available for kidney stones? Which do you suspect Tom would receive?*

Concept Map Exercise

Drawing on what you have learned and studied in Chapter 16, fill in the missing terms in the concept map below.

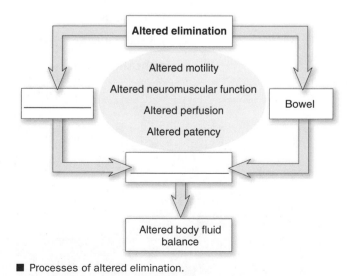

■ Processes of altered elimination.

Chapter 17

Degenerative Changes in Aging

KEY TERMS

accumulated mutations theory

akinesia

amyloid precursor protein (APP)

antagonistic pleiotropy theory

antiresorptive

basal ganglia

β-amyloid protein

bradykinepsia

calcitonin

cellular senescence

chondrocalcinosis

deep brain stimulation (DBS)

developmental theories

1,25-dihydroxycholecal-ciferol

dual energy X-ray absorptiometry (DEXA)

free radical theory

immune senescence

immunologic theory of aging

kyphosis

Lewy body

lipofuscin

menopausal bone loss

neurofibrillary tangles

neuroendocrine theory

osteopenia

osteoporosis

pallidotomy

parathyroid hormone (PTH)

sarcopenia

senescent bone loss

senile plaque

somatic mutation theory

stochastic theories

Chapter Review

1. Aging cells contain a fatty brown lipid pigment that causes stiffening or rigidity. This is known as:

   a. Cellular senescence

   b. Free radical accumulation

   c. Somatic mutation

   d. Lipofuscin

2. As Ron ages, he will have a change in his body mass. He will have a(n) _____ in muscle and a(n) _____ in fat.

   a. Decrease, increase

   b. Increase, decrease

   c. Decrease, decrease

   d. Increase, increase

3. Evelyn has osteopenia. This means that she has:

   a. Lack of white blood cells

   b. Lack of bone marrow

   c. Atrophy of skeletal tissue

   d. Reduced calcification and skeletal bone mass

4. Barb is over age 50 and menopausal. You are counseling her about osteoporosis and tell her that it causes atrophy of the skeletal tissue. Osteoporosis is concerning because it:

   a. Increases the risk for injury due to falls

   b. Causes hypercalcification of the bones

   c. Decreases white blood cell production

   d. Causes sarcopenia

5. Barb has experienced some bone loss already as evidenced by an exaggerated anterior concave curvature of the thoracic spine. This is called:

   a. Senescent bone loss

   b. Kyphosis

   c. Scoliosis

   d. Sarcopenia

6. Causes of sarcopenia include all of the following except:

   a. Limited immune response

   b. Decreased physical activity

   c. Changes in the nervous system

   d. Protein undernutrition

7. A hormone produced by the parathyroid, thyroid, and thymus glands promotes the deposition of calcium and phosphate in bone. This hormone is called:

   a. Estrogen

   b. PTH

   c. Chondrocalcinosis

   d. Calcitonin

8. Because of the alterations that occur in the kidneys due to aging, individuals must be conscious of the types and amounts of medications that they take because the excretion of these medications may be impaired. This increases the individual's risk for:

   a. Shortened duration of medication

   b. Delayed onset of medication

   c. Water intoxification

   d. Drug toxicity

9. The most common type of bone disease affecting older Americans is:

   a. Osteoporosis

   b. Osteopenia

   c. Sarcopenia

   d. Kyphosis

10. Osteoclasts do the following:

    a. Resorb bone

    b. Build bone

    c. Increase calcium uptake

    d. Decease calcium uptake

11. Parkinson disease affects the neurons in the:

    a. Substantia nigra

    b. Cerebrum

    c. Cortex

    d. Brain stem

12. Don has Parkinson disease. He experiences slow movement. This is called:

    a. Akinesia

    b. Bradykinesia

    c. Polykinesia

    d. Kinesia

13. John has Alzheimer disease. Which finding is characteristic of Alzheimer disease:

    a. Kyphosis

    b. Lewy bodies

    c. Neurofibrillary tangles

    d. Intentional tremors

14. Before determining the diagnosis of Alzheimer disease, the provider will rule out all other possible causes. This is called a diagnosis of:

    a. Integration

    b. Evaluation

    c. Inclusion

    d. Exclusion

Case Study 17.1

Don has Parkinson disease. Previous to being diagnosed with Parkinson disease, Don enjoyed biking and jogging. He ate a balanced diet and did not take any unnecessary medication. He has two sisters and one aunt with Parkinson disease. He is 60 years old and currently lives with his wife in their apartment. His wife states that it is becoming very difficult to care for Don at home. Don has had four falls this past month and has been hospitalized once for aspiration pneumonia.

1. Describe the alteration occurring within Don's body. What body processes are affected?

2. What is the most likely cause of Don's Parkinson disease? How did it develop? What risk factors did Don have?

3. *Consider the altered body processes related to the Parkinson disease. What types of complications will occur? What complications is Don experiencing?*

4. *What clinical manifestations would you expect to see with Parkinson disease?*

5. *What current treatment methodologies are available?*

◪ Concept Map Exercise

Drawing on what you have learned and studied in Chapter 17, fill in the missing terms in the concept map below.

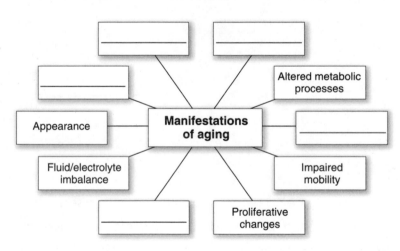

■ Manifestations of aging.

Chapter 18

Combining Complex Pathophysiologic Concepts: Diabetes Mellitus

KEY TERMS

dawn phenomenon

diabetes mellitus

endocrine pancreas

exocrine pancreas

hyperglycemia

hyperketonemia

hypoglycemia

insulin

intermittent claudication

islets of Langerhans

ketoacidosis

Kussmaul respirations

nephropathy

neuropathy

nocturia

polydipsia

polyphagia

polyuria

retinopathy

Somogyi effect

Chapter Review

1. An anabolic hormone required for the uptake of glucose by the many cells is called:

   a. Insulin

   b. Estrogen

   c. Alpha hormone

   d. Beta hormone

2. Todd is a diabetic. He often experiences hyperglycemia. This means:

   a. A decrease in blood glucose

   b. An increase in insulin production

   c. Reabsorption of glucose

   d. Significant elevation in blood glucose

3. Mary has diabetes. She has an absolute or significant deficit of insulin from the destruction of beta cells in the pancreas. Mary has:

   a. Hypoglycemia

   b. Type 3 diabetes

   c. Type 1 diabetes

   d. Type 2 diabetes

4. The three manifestations that are associated with diabetes include all of the following except:

   a. Polyglycemia

   b. Polydipsia

   c. Polyuria

   d. Polyphagia

5. The main goal of treatment for diabetes is to:

   a. Increase episodes of hypoglycemia

   b. Stabilize the blood sugar

   c. Stabilize the immune system

   d. Monitor for infection

6. Thomas, your friend, has been diagnosed with diabetes. He tells you that he has reduced tissue sensitivity to insulin. Thomas most likely has:

   a. Hypoglycemia

   b. Type 3 diabetes

   c. Type 1 diabetes

   d. Type 2 diabetes

7. In type 2 diabetes, the clinical manifestations are:

   a. Acute and nonspecific

   b. Insidious and nonspecific

   c. Acute in nature

   d. Insidious and specific

8. Initial treatment of type 2 diabetes in a patient with a blood sugar of 120 mg/dL will most likely include all of the following except:

   a. Immediate insulin therapy

   b. Diet modification

   c. Exercise

   d. Oral glycemic agents

9. Glucose intolerance that occurs during pregnancy is called:

   a. Glucose resistance

   b. Type 2 diabetes

   c. Type 1 diabetes

   d. Gestational diabetes

10. Mandy has hypoglycemia. You would expect to see all of the following clinical manifestations except:

    a. Hot, dry skin

    b. Pallor

    c. Cool, clammy skin

    d. Weakness

11. The above clinical manifestations that Mandy is experiencing are most likely a result of:

    a. The stress response

    b. Parasympathetic nervous system activation

    c. Sympathetic nervous system activation

    d. Neuronal deprivation of glucose

12. In a patient with type 1 diabetes, severe hyperglycemia (over 400 mg/dL) with deficient insulin can lead to:

    a. Increased production of insulin

    b. Clammy skin

    c. Diabetic ketoacidosis

    d. Weakness

13. During diabetic ketoacidosis, the individual will experience Kussmaul respirations. This occurs because:

    a. The alveoli have collapsed

    b. The body is trying to rid itself of excess acids

    c. There is a decrease in O_2 diffusion

    d. They are short of breath

14. The chronic complications that occur with diabetes are primarily related to:

    a. Episodes of hypoglycemia related to treatment

    b. The stress response

    c. The Somogyi effect

    d. Degenerative changes in the tissues caused by hyperglycemia

15. Karen develops the complication of neuropathy. Neuropathy is:

    a. Nerve degeneration resulting in delayed nerve conduction and impaired sensory function

    b. Shrinking of the nerve cells

    c. Malfunction of the dendrites

    d. Excessive stimulation of the nerve cells

Case Study 18.1

Tony is a 60-year-old obese male who has had type 2 diabetes for 15 years. Prior to his diagnosis, he led a sedentary lifestyle and did not eat a balanced diet. He has an uncle and a cousin with diabetes. His current treatment plan includes oral hypoglycemic medication, diet modification, and an exercise program. Tony has noticed that he is having increased vision problems and has to see his optometrist more frequently. Tony also noticed that the sore on his foot took a very long time to heal. His fasting blood sugar levels have been running 175 to 225 mg/dL over the past month.

1. *Describe the alteration occurring within Tony's body. What body processes are affected?*

2. *What is the most likely cause of Tony's diabetes? How did it develop? What risk factors did Tony have?*

3. *What types of chronic complications occur with diabetes? What complications is Tony experiencing?*

4. *What clinical manifestations would you expect to see with type 2 diabetes? Relate these to Question 1.*

5. *Are the long-term complications of types 1, 2, and gestational diabetes the same? Why or why not?*

▨ Concept Map Exercise

Drawing on what you have learned and studied in Chapter 18, fill in the missing terms in the concept map below.

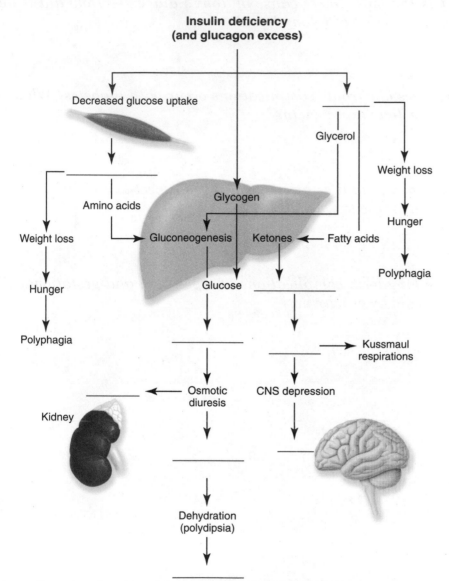

**Insulin deficiency
(and glucagon excess)**

Decreased glucose uptake

Glycerol

Weight loss

Amino acids

Glycogen

Weight loss

Hunger

Gluconeogenesis

Ketones ← Fatty acids

Hunger

Polyphagia

Glucose

Polyphagia

Kussmaul
respirations

Kidney

Osmotic
diuresis

CNS depression

Dehydration
(polydipsia)

■ Mechanisms of hyperglycemia and hyperketonemia. CNS, central nervous system.

Answer Key

CHAPTER 1 INTRODUCTION TO PATHOPHYSIOLOGY

CHAPTER REVIEW

1. a

2. b

3. Epidemiology allows us to understand disease through the identification of its patterns and causes. It also helps us understand how to control the disease and apply the three levels of prevention.

4. b

5. c

6. Gender, age, race, locale, socioeconomic factors, and ethnicity.

7. b

8. d

9. a

10. a

11. b

12. b

13. c

14. b

15. Prevention is associated with stopping the onset or progression of a disease, whereas intervention is a specific action taken in relation to the treatment of the disease itself or the human response related to the alteration caused by the disease.

16. c

17. a

18. b

19. a

20. Answers will vary.

CASE STUDY 1.1

1. Alteration in oxygenation/tissue perfusion.
2. Inactivity, obesity, and history of smoking. Yes, these can be modified.
3. Most likely, Aubre's gender did play a part in the delay of diagnosis and treatment of the myocardial infarction. This, however, is changing as more and more health care providers are aware of gender bias in terms of research and patient

care. The individualized approach to the management of the human response to an alteration in health can include the following: increased cultural awareness/competency, awareness of gender bias, and collaboration.

4. The cells are deprived of oxygen. This will initially alter their ability to function and ultimately cause cellular death.

5. The cells will change their metabolism from an aerobic state to an anaerobic state.

6. Typical signs and symptoms would be chest pain and/or discomfort, shortness of breath, paleness, nausea, and shoulder pain.

CONCEPT MAP EXERCISE

Consult Figure 1.1 (Concept map. Pathophysiology terms) on p. 4 of the textbook to check your answers.

CHAPTER 2 ALTERED CELLS AND TISSUES

CHAPTER REVIEW

1. d
2. c
3. d
4. a
5. a
6. d
7. a
8. b
9. b
10. c
11. d
12. d
13. a
14. b
15. b

CASE STUDY 2.1

1. Answers will vary with each student's viewpoint. Some people identify illness as part of the cycle of life and anticipate times of illness and alteration within the body. Others view health and illness on opposite ends of a continuum. A person's definition of health and illness depends upon a number of variables such as their culture, past experiences with alterations in health (chronic illness), and their beliefs and values.

2. Tom probably viewed his status as healthy because, as he said, he didn't "feel sick." Many individuals like Tom define their health in terms of being able to meet their daily commitments. Tom definitely does have some alterations in his health status. Although these alterations may not seem acute, they do affect Tom's total health.

3. The melanoma cell can spread to adjacent cells and tissues, causing a change in cellular function. The melanoma can disrupt homeostasis as it affects groups of cells (tissues) and then organs. This will lead to adaptations within the organ to a point that it may not be able to function. This organ dysfunction will lead to a disruption in homeostasis within the body.

4. and 5. Consult Figure 2.4 (Adaptive cell changes. Normal cells adapt to stress by altering size, number, or type/structure.) on p. 15 of the textbook to check your drawing of each type of cell change.
   - **Hypertrophy:** Cells enlarge, cause enlargement of tissues/organs.

Reversible when signal stimulating the enlargement is removed. An example of this would be uterine enlargement during pregnancy.

- **Hyperplasia:** An increase in the number of cells. Reversible when signal stimulating the enlargement is removed. An example of this would be uterine enlargement during pregnancy.
- **Metaplasia:** Changing of one cell type to another; leads to cell adaptation. Often reversible if cellular stressor is removed.
- **Dysplasia:** The actual change in cell size, shape, uniformity, arrangement, and structure. Low-grade dysplasia is potentially reversible. High-grade dysplasia is not, because it cannot be differentiated from in situ carcinoma.
- **Atrophy:** The decrease in the size of a cell. Atrophy may or may not be reversible, depending on the cells involved. Atrophy from muscle disuse can be reversed by resuming exercise. However, in instances where blood supply is compromised or nerve cells are damaged, atrophy reversal is less likely. The reversibility of atrophy also depends on the cause of the atrophy (e.g., poor nutrition, aging, inadequate blood perfusion, inactivity).

CASE STUDY 2.2

1. Irregular menses with heavier bleeding at times. Vaginal dryness, fatigue, disrupted sleep patterns, and mood swings. Changes in FSH and estradiol blood levels.
2. Increased FSH levels (normal premenopausal range: 5 to 30 IU/L; common postmenopausal range: >30 IU/L) and decreased estradiol levels (normal premenopausal range: 20 to 400 pg/mL; common postmenopausal range: 2 to 25 pg/mL). These changes occur because initially reduced release of ovarian hormones causes stimulation of the anterior pituitary with increasing secretion of FSH and LH.
3. There is a decrease in the trophic stimulation of the hormones associated with ovarian cycles. This decrease in hormonal stimulation is the catalyst for the alterations that occur within the cells, resulting in the menopausal signs and symptoms experienced by the individual. The body responds by the alteration of cells within the following organs: breasts, kidneys, endometrium, ovaries, and vagina.
4. Answers and concept maps will vary, but should include the following:
   - **Dyspareunia:** Thinning of the skin and lack of lubrication, which can alter sexual response.
   - **Hot flashes or flushes:** Vasomotor symptoms associated with menopause; likely the result of altered thermoregulation.
   - **Bone demineralization:** Resulting from the effects of cytokines in the absence of the protective effects of the ovarian hormones.
   - **Altered sexual functioning:** Resulting from decreased level of circulating hormones and the changes that take place with the vagina (thinning of vaginal walls, decreased lubrication).
   - **Metrorrhagia:** Irregular intervals between menses due to changes in the hormonal levels.
5. Answers will vary, but may include the following:
   - Offer the opportunity for her husband to accompany her on her next visit to discuss the changes occurring within her body.
   - Provide her with educational materials such as pamphlets and handouts.

ACTIVITY

¹S	²I	G	³N			⁴S	Y	M	⁵P	T	O	M		⁶P		⁷S
	A		O			T			I				⁸R	⁹R	I	S	K
	¹⁰T	I	S	S	U	E		¹¹I	N	C	I	D	E	N	C	E			I
	R		O			R		O					A	¹²V	E	I	N
	O		¹³C	H	R	O	N	I	C					A	
	G		O			I			Y		¹⁴M	E	T	A	P	L	A	¹⁵S	I	¹⁶A
	E		¹⁷A	D	A	P	T				E			H		P
	N		I			¹⁸O	X	Y	¹⁹G	E	N		N		O		O
	I		A		²⁰N		S		R			C		C		P
²¹C	²²E	L	²³L		²⁴E	T	I	O	L	O	G	Y	E		K		T
	N		O		C		S		W				²⁵H		O
	Z		C		R			²⁶T	H	E	²⁷R	M	A	L		S
	Y		²⁸A	T	R	O	P	H	Y		O		I		I
	M		L		²⁹S						²⁹S	T	R	E	³⁰S	S
	E			³¹I	M	M	U	N	E				K
³²O	S	M	O	S	I	S					³³G	O	L	G	I

CHAPTER 3 INFLAMMATION AND TISSUE REPAIR

CHAPTER REVIEW

1. b
2. e
3. a
4. d
5. c
6. c
7. e
8. c
9. d
10. a
11. e
12. b
13. b
14. d
15. d
16. a
17. c
18. b
19. a
20. b

CASE STUDY 3.1

1.
- **Vascular Response:** Occurs immediately after tissue injury. This response involves the release of chemical mediators that control vascular permeability leading to increased blood flow to the area. The vascular response includes activation of the complement system (source of chemical mediators).
- **Cellular Response:** Cells required for tissue healing and repair respond to the injury. The steps involved include: chemotaxis, cellular adherence, and cellular migration.

The catalyst or trigger for the acute inflammatory response is the tissue injury.

2. Yes. This type of burn will damage the epidermal skin layers and penetrate some dermal skin layers. As long as the nerve cells are intact, Brian will feel the sensation of pain.

3. Brian would experience pain, redness, edema, and loss of function of the affected area. These clinical manifestations are due to the vascular and cellular responses occurring within his body. Also, depending on the size of the burns, there might be large fluid shifts within the body due to the increase in the vascular permeability.

4. The wounds will heal by secondary intention. Increased blood supply to the area assists with the formation of granulation tissue within the wound bed. If the burn is superficial, the new tissue will gradually fill in the area. If necrosis of the tissue occurs in the upper epidermal layers, scarring is avoided. However, if tissue necrosis occurs in both epidermal and upper dermal layers, collagen will fill in the wound bed and lead to scarring.

5. Dressing changes with wound débridement and analgesics to manage the pain. Skin grafting would be an option as well, depending on the depth of the burn.

6. Complications include:
- The release of large amounts of chemical mediators can cause fluid shifts due to the vascular permeability. The fluid will shift from the vascular space into the interstitial space.
- To heal wounds, the body requires a large amount of energy and the metabolism will increase drastically. If the body's increased metabolic needs are not met, the following could occur: tissue hypoxia, tissue wasting, and infection.
- The skin is considered as the first line of defense. When the integrity of the skin is impaired, microbes can easily enter the body.

CASE STUDY 3.2

1. Acute inflammation will resolve within a fairly short period of time. Chronic inflammation occurs over a period of time and may cause alteration of the cells/tissues due to the prolonged stressors placed on those cells. These alterations can result in functional changes within the tissue.

2. Local changes occur within the joints in a symmetrical fashion. Clinical manifestations include: erythema, pain, swelling, warmth, and decreased mobility. Over time, changes occur within the joints causing malalignment or deviation of the joints.

3. Due to the chronic inflammation in the joints, destruction of the tissue will occur. Because of the tissue destruction, Terri will experience an alteration of the normal function in her joints and will not have the flexion and extension capabilities. Systemic response to the chronic inflammation includes: fever, fatigue, anemia, anorexia, weight loss, and weakness. Also, consider the fact that chronic pain can also lead to situational depression.

4. Joint destruction over time will cause joint malalignment and deviation.

This would make it difficult for Terri to perform even simple activities such as combing her hair, brushing her teeth, or driving her car.

5. In response to the systemic alterations that occur with rheumatoid arthritis such as anemia, compensation will occur due to the low hemoglobin. The body will respond as follows: increased respiration rate and increased heart rate. The body is attempting to maintain homeostasis by increasing the supply of oxygen (increased respiration) and moving it around the body faster (increased heart rate).

6. Pain, decreased ability to care for one-self, decreased ability to participate fully in activities that you may enjoy.

CONCEPT MAP EXERCISE

Consult Figure 3.3 (Concept map. An overview of the importance of chemical mediators in the vascular and cellular responses of inflammation.) on p. 37, Figure 3.4 (Concept map. An example of one mechanism of the interrelationship between the clotting, complement, and kinin systems: activation of clotting factor XII) on p. 39, Figure 3.5. (Concept map. Phases of healing and tissue repair.) on p. 42, and Figure 3.12 (Concept map. The process of chronic inflammation leading to granuloma formation.) on p. 49 of the textbook to check your answers.

CHAPTER 4   ALTERED IMMUNITY

CHAPTER REVIEW

1. d
2. d
3. b
4. c
5. a
6. d
7. b
8. c
9. c
10. b
11. c
12. a
13. a
14. b
15. d

CASE STUDY 4.1

1. SLE is an autoimmune disease that includes the type III hypersensitivity reaction of antigen–antibody complex deposition stimulating an inflammatory response. In the type III response, autoantibodies are targeted against the self. The immune system is unable to distinguish self from nonself, producing autoantibodies by plasma cells and cytotoxic T cells that target self. The inflammation stimulated by complex deposition can cause permanent organ and tissue damage.

2. Andrea has a rash on her cheeks. She also complains of pain in her joints in her fingers as well as fatigue. These manifestations are due to the inflammation induced by complex deposition. This inflammation is chronic in nature. The chronic inflammation will cause structural and functional changes over time. The laboratory findings reflect the autoimmune response against nuclear components in the cell.

3. It is important for the body to be able to identify itself because of the way the immune system operates. If the body is unable to differentiate between self and nonself, it runs the risk of attacking its own cells and tissues.

4. Treatments designed to reduce activity of the immune response:

- DMARDS: disease-modifying anti-rheumatoid drugs
- Nonsteroidal anti-inflammatory drugs
- Corticosteroids

Effects: delay the progress and resulting damage with anti-rheumatoid drugs.

CASE STUDY 4.2

1. Components of healthy immune system:
   - Innate immunity
   - Adaptive immunity: specificity, diversity, memory, self, and nonself recognition
   - Humoral immunity
   - Cell-mediated immunity

   Alterations within immune system in an individual with AIDS:
   - Immunosuppression
   - Loss of CD4 T cells
   - Loss of cell-mediated immunity
   - Loss of humoral immunity

2. Increases susceptibility to many common pathogens resulting in severe infections. The individual will also have an increased number of infections. This is due to the loss of cell-mediated and humoral immunity. The clinical manifestations (both local and systemic) are due to the infections present within the body as well as the decreased capability to deal with the infections.

3. Trish's immune system is suppressed. Because of the loss of CD4 T cells, her body is not able to actively respond to infections that enter her body. Because of the HIV, she is also at an increased risk for certain types of cancer and opportunistic infections.

4. Treatments:
   - Antiretroviral agents to target the virus
   - Highly active antiretroviral therapy (HAART)
   - Counseling

   The treatments for HIV and AIDS are similar. Treatment for individuals with HIV is aimed at keeping their CD4 T cells at an optimum level. Treatment for individuals with AIDS is primarily aimed at controlling the opportunistic infections present and increasing the CD4 T cells. At the point the individual develops AIDS, the immune system is severely compromised. Identification of patients as being HIV positive means that they have the virus and must be monitored very closely for the progression into AIDS. As individuals progress from HIV to AIDS, the CD4 T cells will decline and the episodes of infections will increase.

CONCEPT MAP EXERCISE

Consult Figure 4.1 (Concept map. Cellular components involved in immune defense) on p. 69 of the textbook to check your answers.

CHAPTER 5 INFECTION

CHAPTER REVIEW

1. d
2. a
3. c
4. b
5. a
6. a
7. d
8. b
9. c
10. b
11. d
12. b
13. a
14. c
15. b
16. c
17. d

18. b

19. a

20. b

21. b

22. c

23. a

24. b

25. b

CASE STUDY 5.1

1. Virus. The respiratory epithelial cells are armed with cilia, mucus, and antibodies. The influenza virus impairs these protections. The virus causes infected epithelial cell death resulting in necrosis and sloughing of the dead cells. Loss of protections can lead to bacterial pneumonia, a common complication of influenza. When infection is found in the lungs, this leads to cell death and sloughing of alveolar lining cells.
2. Yes; influenza viruses gradually change genetic composition during replication in the human host cell in a process called reassortment. This process results in a virus that has genetic modification. The result is that, because the virus changes from year to year, one must receive the vaccination each year.
3. Close living quarters make it easier to pass the virus from person to person. Also, elderly may have chronic conditions that may increase their susceptibility to the virus.
4. Have her receive a vaccination prior to the influenza season and teach her about universal precautions.
5. Isolation for those with the virus; cough and cover; stay 3 feet away from the infected individual; encourage healthy lifestyle to maintain host defenses.

CONCEPT MAP EXERCISE

Consult Figure 5.10 (Concept map. Phases of infection and corresponding clinical manifestations) on p. 111 and Figure 5.13 (Concept map. Alterations in liver function and manifestations of liver failure) on p. 117 of the textbook to check your answers.

ACTIVITY: A COMPARISON OF COMMON PATHOGENS

Pathogen	Unique Structure Characteristics	Replication	Toxin Production	Treatment Measures
Bacteria	Complex outer cell wall	Does not require human host to reproduce; bacteria divide by binary fission	Yes; some bacteria produce toxins	Antibiotics/ Antibacterials
Viruses	Protein coat and a core of either DNA or RNA	Requires living host cell for replication	No	Treat symptoms; antivirals may be effective in reducing time of infection if initiated at onset
Fungi	Hyphae intertwine to form mycelium	Budding, extension of hyphae, or producing spores	No	Antifungals
Protozoa	Highly diverse; unicellular	Variable; some reproduce by binary fission or conjugation (two join and exchange genetic material)	No; some may secrete enzymes that cause tissue destruction	Variable; antibiotics may be effective in some cases

CHAPTER 6 GENETIC AND DEVELOPMENTAL DISORDERS

CHAPTER REVIEW

1. a
2. b
3. d
4. d
5. a
6. b
7. d
8. c
9. c
10. b
11. d
12. c
13. a
14. d
15. b

CASE STUDY 6.1

1. The genetic mutation is located on chromosome 11. The mutated gene directly affects the production of the hemoglobin resulting in production of hemoglobin S. Because of this gene mutation, the hemoglobin's shape will be changed into a sickle shape.

2. Sickle cell anemia is an autosomal recessive disorder. People with sickle cell anemia such as Ashland inherit the sickle cell gene from both parents. If Ashland had only one sickle cell gene, he would be a carrier. It is possible that his brother is a carrier. When both parents have the sickle cell trait, there is a one in four (25%) chance that their baby will inherit two mutated genes and have the disease. There is a 50% chance that the baby will inherit one normal gene and one mutated gene.

3. Sickle cell crisis; pain in his legs, back, and arms; fatigue (related to anemia); and frequent infections (related to the damage in the spleen due to the sickle cell disease). The pain arises from the damage that the irregularly shaped hemoglobin is doing at the cellular level. As the sickle-shaped hemoglobin attempts to pass through the micro-circulation, it adheres to other sickled cells and reduces blood flow in the vessel. The irregularly shaped hemoglobin damages the endothelial cells lining blood vessels. It also can damage organs such as the spleen and lungs.

4. Prevention of complications related to infection: immunizations. Supportive care/treatment aimed at symptoms such as pain. Hydroxyurea: to increase the production of hemoglobin F (HbF) (this prevents the formation of HbS).

CASE STUDY 6.2

1. Huntington disease is an autosomal dominant genetic disorder. It is a progressive disorder that affects the neurologic system. The defect is in the huntingtin gene on chromosome 4. This mutation generates a code for the abnormal huntingtin protein.

2. The abnormal protein accumulates and destroys nerve cells. Because of the destruction of nerve cells, the individual will experience involuntary movements, cognitive impairment, personality changes, and loss of memory. The clinical manifestations correlate to nerve cells destroyed (i.e., as the damage progresses to the different nerve cells in the body, the functions that those nerve cells controlled will be altered).

3. With genetic counseling, Lee's children can make an informed decision about the risks of passing on the genetic disorder

to their children. They may or may not decide to have the genetic testing to see if they carry the gene, as there is no treatment for it. Some individuals want to know; others do not.

CHAPTER 7 ALTERED CELLULAR PROLIFERATION AND DIFFERENTIATION

CHAPTER REVIEW

1. a
2. b
3. c
4. c
5. d
6. d
7. a
8. b
9. b
10. d
11. a
12. d
13. c
14. b
15. a

CASE STUDY 7.1

1. There is an increase in cellular proliferation (unregulated growth) and loss of cellular differentiation.
2. *Local:* As the tumor enlarges, it will place pressure on the adjacent tissues causing crowding of the tissues/ organs. The tumor could also cause an obstruction of the colon. Symptoms will vary depending on the location of the tumor. The tumor will also deprive the local tissues of blood flow thereby decreasing the nutrients and oxygen delivered to the local tissues. *Systemic:*

CONCEPT MAP EXERCISE

Consult Figure 6.13 (Concept map. Genetic alterations in human disease) on p. 142 of the textbook to check your answers.

Corrine will experience anemia related to the body's response to the enlarging tumor. Corrine may also experience weight loss (related to the tumor utilizing a large portion of her caloric intake), wasting of muscle, and loss of appetite related to the effects of the tumor.

3. Cancer cells in the colon invade the basement membrane and have access to lymph capillaries. Once the cancer cells enter the lymph system, they have access to lymph nodes, particularly the mesenteric lymph nodes. These same cancer cells may also enter the blood capillaries and then metastasize through the portal circulation to the liver.
4. Surgical excision of the tumor, radiation, and chemotherapy. All of these treatments work in synergy against the cancer.
5. Genetic (both of her brothers have developed colon cancer), age (colon cancer most commonly occurs in individuals over age 50).

CASE STUDY 7.2

1. The enlarging tumor is interfering with the process of ventilation and diffusion.
2. Cough, shortness of breath, chest pain, and fatigue.
3. Relationship between alteration and clinical manifestations:
   - **Chronic cough:** related to the presence of the tumor in the lung

- **Shortness of breath:** related to the tumor compressing alveoli causing impaired oxygen diffusion
- **Chest pain:** related to the enlarging tumor compressing lung tissue
- **Fatigue:** related to the alteration in oxygen diffusion resulting in a decreased amount of oxygen and nutrition carried to the tissues
4. Surgical removal of the tumor, radiation treatment to the tumor area (kills

any cancerous cells left behind), and chemotherapy (targets any cancer cells that may have metastasized in the body).

CONCEPT MAP EXERCISE

Consult Figure 7.2 (Concept map. The genomic mechanisms of cancer) on p. 161 of the textbook to check your answers.

CHAPTER 8 ALTERED FLUID, ELECTROLYTE, AND ACID–BASE BALANCE

CHAPTER REVIEW

1. a
2. d
3. b
4. c
5. a
6. b
7. d
8. a
9. d
10. b
11. c
12. c
13. d
14. c
15. c

CASE STUDY 8.1

1. The alteration in fluid balance resulting in edema is due to increased hydrostatic forces promoting movement of fluid out of the vascular space into the interstitium. Because the heart is not pumping effectively in congestive heart failure, blood is backing up into the venous

system. The increased pressure inside the vessels favors filtration of fluid from the vascular space into the interstitium. Because Lila's feet are "dependent" or lower than her heart, they are more likely to be affected by edema.
2. Lila's condition is associated with hypervolemia. She may also have increased weight gain due to the increase in total body water resulting from the edema she is experiencing. Lila may also develop shortness of breath, due to edema in the lung interstitial tissue called pulmonary edema. Pulmonary edema makes it difficult to exchange gasses, causing problems with oxygenation. Lila may also have difficulty sleeping, since lying flat causes increased blood return to the heart.
3. In addition to treating Lila's primary problem related to heart failure, management of fluid balance can be accomplished with balanced fluid intake and output and use of drugs that would promote fluid loss (i.e., diuretics). Careful attention must also be paid to assure that Lila does not develop an electrolyte imbalance.
4. Since water moves together with sodium, an increase in sodium content in the diet will increase fluid retention and promote edema within the

body. Likewise, when an individual is given a diuretic, the medication works to decrease reabsorption of sodium in the kidney. As this accomplished, more fluid is excreted from the body.

CONCEPT MAP EXERCISE

Consult Figure 8.13 (Concept map. Fluid, electrolyte and acid–base balance) on p. 203 of the textbook to check your answers.

CHAPTER 9 ALTERED NEURONAL TRANSMISSION

CHAPTER REVIEW

1. a
2. d
3. c
4. b
5. a
6. d
7. c
8. b
9. d
10. a
11. d
12. c
13. c
14. d
15. c

CASE STUDY 9.1

1. Altered neuronal transmission. There is a disruption in the neuronal communication due to the degeneration of the myelin.
2. The symptoms/clinical manifestations result from impairment in neurologic transduction.
3. Clinical manifestations include blurred vision, loss of muscle control, and fatigue. Each of the manifestations can be traced back to the degeneration of the myelin of the specific nerves affected.
4. Progressive. Marilyn will most likely experience periods of exacerbation countered with periods of remission of symptoms of the disease as it progresses.

5. Drugs will be prescribed to help modify the disease because there is no cure. The health care team will focus on managing symptoms and slowing the progression of the disease.

CASE STUDY 9.2

1. Congenital, brain tumor, intraventricular hemorrhage, meningitis, and traumatic injury to the head. Congenital.
2. Noncommunicating hydrocephalus: this is due to CSF flow obstruction. Communicating hydrocephalus: this is due to impaired CSF absorption.
3. The system in which the CSF circulates is a closed system. If the amount of fluid is increased, there is no where for it to go. The increased amount of CSF will increase the pressure on the surrounding tissues. Because of the pressure, there will be impaired tissue perfusion, ultimately leading to ischemia and cell death.
4. Clinical manifestations include increased head circumference, irritability, difficulty feeding, and impaired motor and cognitive functions. In Ray, this impaired function may be manifested as a delay in his cognitive and motor development.
5. The shunt will need to be replaced as Ray grows. Ray is at an increased risk for infection due to the shunt.

CONCEPT MAP EXERCISE

Consult Figure 9.15 (Concept map. Mechanisms of neuronal disorders) on p. 235 of the textbook to check your answers.

CHAPTER 10 ALTERED SENSORY FUNCTION AND PAIN PERCEPTION

CHAPTER REVIEW

1. a
2. b
3. d
4. c
5. a
6. d
7. b
8. c
9. d
10. a
11. b
12. c
13. b
14. a
15. d

CASE STUDY 10.1

1. Because of Shane's cold, his eustachian tubes became occluded and fluids/secretions pooled in this area. This warm, moist environment provides an optimal environment for growth of viruses and bacterial pathogens. The infection serves as a catalyst for the inflammation process. Because of the inflammation process, the tympanic membrane as well as the surrounding cells and tissues become edematous and painful. This will impact the normal process of the transmission of sound waves in the ear.
2. The sensation of pain and increased pressure as evidenced by redness (hyperemia), bulging (accumulation of fluid) of the tympanic membrane. Shane refuses to nurse because the sucking action increases the pressure in his eustachian tube, causing increased discomfort. The fever is a manifestation secondary to the immune system response and inflammatory response due to the bacterial pathogen.
3. Observation without the use of antibiotics. If AOM is unresponsive to observation, the use of antibiotics such as Amoxicillin is indicated. The anitbiotic will target the bacterial pathogen. Other supportive measures may be used to decrease pain and inflammation such as the use of ibuprofen.
4. With chronic inflammation, scar tissue will form. If this occurs within the tympanic membrane, hearing loss will ensue due to the build up of scar tissue on the membrane.

CASE STUDY 10.2

1. Glaucoma causes increased intraocular pressure due to the obstruction of the trabecular network (this network normally drains the aqueous humor to help maintain normal pressure within the eye).
2. Age and diabetes.
3. The increased pressure is the catalyst for decreased tissue perfusion to adjacent cells and tissue. This leads to damage to the optic nerve in the posterior eye. Eventually, if the pressure remains high, Ruby will lose her sight.
4. Initially, primary open angle glaucoma has no symptoms. This is why routine screening is so important. As it progresses, the individual will experience vision loss due to the increased pressure on the optic nerve.
5. Treatments are targeted at decreasing the intraocular pressure. Types of treatments include: medications to decrease the fluid production and

increase the outflow of fluid; surgery to correct the trabecular network or increase fluid outflow.

CONCEPT MAP EXERCISE

Consult Figure 10.14 (Concept map. Sensory alterations) to check your answers.

CHAPTER 11 ALTERED HORMONAL AND METABOLIC REGULATION

CHAPTER REVIEW

1. c
2. b
3. d
4. a
5. c
6. a
7. a
8. b
9. c
10. a
11. a
12. d
13. a
14. d
15. b

3. Recall the immune system and the concept of antibodies/antigens. In Graves disease, autoantibodies directed toward the TSH receptor of the thyroid trigger increased stimulation of the thyroid gland. This leads to increased secretion of thyroid hormones and enlargement of the thyroid gland.
4. Weight loss, restlessness, heat intolerance, exophthalmos, and enlarged thyroid. You will see systemic and local effect from the alteration. Systemically, Donna's metabolism is increased (resulting in weight loss). Locally, Donna experiences exophthalmos related to the interaction of TSH-sensitized antibodies interacting with fibroblast antigens found in extraocular muscles and tissues.
5. TSH levels, serum-free thyroxine level, serum T3 and T4, and radioactive iodine test.

CASE STUDY 11.1

1. There is a hyperstimulation of the thyroid gland related to an autoimmune response.
2. Autoimmune, gender, and environmental factors.

CONCEPT MAP EXERCISE

Consult Figure 11.7 (Concept map. Stress pathways) on p. 288 of the textbook to check your answers.

CHAPTER 12 ALTERED REPRODUCTIVE FUNCTION

CHAPTER REVIEW

1. a
2. d
3. c
4. a

5. b
6. a
7. d
8. b
9. a

10. b

11. a

12. b

13. c

14. a

15. b

16. a

17. a

18. d

19. b

CASE STUDY 12.1

1. Irregular menses with heavier bleeding at times. Vaginal dryness, fatigue, disrupted sleep patterns, and mood swings. Changes in FSH and estradiol blood levels.
2. Increased FSH levels (normal premenopausal range: 5 to 30 IU/L; common postmenopausal range: >30 IU/L) and decreased estradiol levels (normal premenopausal range: 20 to 400 pg/ml; common postmenopausal range: 2 to 25 pg/mL). These changes occur because initially reduced release of ovarian hormones causes stimulation of the anterior pituitary with increasing secretion of FSH and LH.
3. There is a decrease in the trophic stimulation of the hormones associated with ovarian cycles. This decrease in hormonal stimulation is the catalyst for the alterations that occur within the cells, resulting in the menopausal signs and symptoms experienced by the individual. The body responds by the alteration of cells within the following organs: breasts, kidneys, endometrium, ovaries, and vagina.
4. Answers and concept maps will vary, but should include:
   * *Dyspareunia:* thinning of the skin and lack of lubrication, which can alter sexual response.
   * *Hot flashes or flushes:* vasomotor symptoms associated with menopause; likely the result of altered thermoregulation.
   * *Bone demineralization:* resulting from the effects of cytokines in the absence of the protective effects of the ovarian hormones.
   * *Altered sexual functioning:* resulting from decreased level of circulating hormones and the changes that take place with the vagina (thinning of vaginal walls, decreased lubrication).
   * *Metrorrhagia:* irregular intervals between menses due to changes in the hormonal levels.
5. Answers will vary, but may include:
   * Offer the opportunity for her husband to accompany her on her next visit to discuss the changes occurring within her body.
   * Provide her with educational materials such as pamphlets and handouts.

CONCEPT MAP EXERCISE

Consult Figure 12.14 (Concept map. Pathogenesis of polycystic ovary syndrome.) on p. 313 of the textbook to check your answers.

CHAPTER 13   ALTERED VENTILATION AND DIFFUSION

CHAPTER REVIEW

1. d
2. b
3. c
4. a
5. a
6. a
7. b

8. c

9. d

10. a

11. b

12. a

13. d

14. c

15. c

CASE STUDY 13.1

1. The inflammatory and immune responses are triggered secondary to invasion of a pathogen. The inflamed alveoli fill with exudates and other products of inflammation accumulate as well. This causes consolidation of the lung tissue, thus altering the process of diffusion.

2. Etiology: Bacterial, viral, and fungal infectious agents.

- Risk factors: Age and chronic respiratory disease process (asthma).
- Expected course: Infection will resolve with treatment of antibiotics and supportive care.

3. Alterations in ventilation and diffusion. The pneumonia causes accumulation of exudates in the alveoli, decreasing the surface area for diffusion of oxygen.

4. Cough (local), fever (systemic), shortness of breath (local), and chest pain (local).

5. Antibiotics to target the pathogen. Supportive measures include: increase fluid intake, medication to reduce fever and discomfort, and use of supplemental oxygen.

CONCEPT MAP EXERCISE

Consult Figure 13.2 (Concept map. Altered ventilation and diffusion) on p. 336 of the textbook to check your answers.

CHAPTER 14 ALTERED PERFUSION

CHAPTER REVIEW

1. d

2. a

3. a

4. d

5. d, a, b, e, c

6. c

7. a

8. b

9. d

10. d

11. a

12. a

13. a

14. b

15. d

CASE STUDY 14.1

1. Altered perfusion and altered diffusion of oxygen. Meriam's cardiac output is decreased and tissue perfusion is decreased.

2. *Fluid weight gain:* Related to altered perfusion, especially perfusion of the kidneys.
   Cough: Increased fluid collection in the lungs.
   Shortness of breath: Decreased O_2 diffusion due to the fluid accumulation in the lungs.

3. Most likely related to diabetes, obesity, and hypertension.

4. The development of Meriam's heart failure is most likely related to her chronic co-morbid conditions of diabetes and hypertension. The heart is one of the target organs that diabetes affects over time. If Meriam's hypertension is uncontrolled over time, her heart must work harder to pump against the peripheral resistance. This will ultimately cause hypertrophy of the cardiac muscle, causing it to be less efficient.

5. Supplemental oxygen, diuretics to get rid of the extra fluid, possibly medications to increase her cardiac output and strengthen the heart contraction.

CASE STUDY 14.2

1. Neurologic system functioning is altered. Brain cells lack O_2 and are unable to function properly. If deprived of O_2 long enough, irreversible cellular damage and death will occur.

2. Plaque builds up in the arteries (narrowing the lumen) due to the high cholesterol, smoking contributes to arteriosclerosis (vessels not as pliable), and long standing hypertension leads to vessel damage.

3. Roman was dizzy with slurred speech and mouth drooping. The clinical manifestations observed correlate to the part of the brain that is injured.

4. The left side.

5. CT scan. Treatment is aimed at removing the clot or stopping the bleeding in the brain. Treatment also focuses on reducing cerebral edema.

CONCEPT MAP EXERCISE

Consult Figure 14.8 (Concept map. Altered perfusion) on p. 368 of the textbook to check your answers.

CHAPTER 15   ALTERED NUTRITION

CHAPTER REVIEW

1. d
2. a
3. c
4. a
5. b
6. c
7. d
8. e
9. a
10. c
11. d
12. b
13. c
14. b
15. c

CASE STUDY 15.1

1. Alteration in absorption. Celiac disease is a disorder of gluten malabsorption. It is due to a T cell–mediated hypersensitivity to gluten in persons who are genetically predisposed to develop this condition. Absorption is also impaired as these villi undergo atrophy.

2. Connie does not identify any familial history of celiac disease. This does not mean that it is not present. Many individuals with celiac disease do not know that they have it. However, Connie is of Western European heritage; a group with a high prevalence of this disease.

3. The chronic irritation of the gastrointestinal lining can cause inflammatory and atrophic tissue changes (remember metaplasia, dysplasia?). Damage to the intestinal mucosa inhibits digestion due to damage to the villi. Connie is experiencing bloating and abdominal discomfort.

4. Weight loss, diarrhea, steatorrhea, malodorous stools, abdominal bloating, fatigue, and nutritional and vitamin deficiencies.

5. Test serum for antibodies and small bowel biopsy.

CONCEPT MAP EXERCISE

Consult Figure 15.7 (Concept map. Altered Nutrition) on p. 405 of the textbook to check your answers.

CHAPTER 16 ALTERED ELIMINATION

CHAPTER REVIEW

1. a
2. b
3. c
4. d
5. c
6. a
7. c
8. d
9. c
10. a
11. b
12. b
13. a
14. b
15. d

2. The stones could be related to his increased calcium oxalate intake. Kidney stones form from elevated urinary levels of calcium and stasis from urinary filtrate may promote development of the stones. Tom's risk factors include a diet with foods high in calcium oxalate.

3. Inflammation, infection, and obstruction.

4. Severe flank pain due to the presence of stone in the tissue.

5. Pain management, hydration, and removal of the stone. Tom would receive lithotripsy, percutaneous nephrolithotomy, and ureteroscopic stone removal.

CONCEPT MAP EXERCISE

Consult Figure 16.11 (Concept map. Processes of altered elimination) on p. 438 of the textbook to check your answers.

CASE STUDY 16.1

1. Alteration in elimination. Tom's kidneys are not able to function normally due to the presence of stone.

CHAPTER 17   DEGENERATIVE CHANGES IN AGING

CHAPTER REVIEW

1. d
2. a
3. c
4. a
5. b
6. a
7. d
8. d
9. a
10. a
11. a
12. b
13. c
14. d

CASE STUDY 17.1

1. There is degeneration of the nigrostriatal pathway leading to reduction in the neurotransmitter, dopamine. Because of the lack of dopamine, Don has difficulty getting his body to do what his brain is telling it to do. Don will experience bradykinesia and other neurological symptoms.
2. There seems to be a familial inheritance pattern with the Parkinson in Don's family. No other risk factors noted.
3. Complications related to decreased mobility/activity and decreased muscle control. Don experienced falls related to the decreased mobility and aspiration due to the dysphagia.
4. Tremor, rigidity, bradykinesia, and postural instability.
5. *Pharmacological:* Sinemet, dopamine agonists.
   Surgical: Pallidotomy and deep brain stimulation.

CONCEPT MAP EXERCISE

Consult Figure 17.3 (Concept map. Manifestations of aging) on p. 454 of the textbook to check your answers.

CHAPTER 18   COMBINING COMPLEX PATHOPHYSIOLOGIC CONCEPTS: DIABETES MELLITUS

CHAPTER REVIEW

1. a
2. d
3. c
4. a
5. b
6. d
7. b
8. a
9. d
10. a
11. d
12. c
13. b
14. d
15. a

CASE STUDY 18.1

1. Alteration in the endocrine system and lack of insulin production coupled with insulin resistance in the cells.

Metabolism is affected, wound healing is slow, etc.

2. Tony has the risk factors for type 2 diabetes: obesity, sedentary lifestyle, and poor diet. The combination of these factors most likely contributed to the alteration that occurred in his body.

3. Microvascular and macrovascular complications including neuropathy, retinopathy, and heart and kidney damage. Tony is currently experiencing retinopathy.

4. Fatigue, hyperglycemia, visual changes, changes in kidney function, coronary artery disease, peripheral vascular disease, recurrent infections, or neuropathy.

5. Yes, all types of diabetes increase the blood sugar which is the catalyst for degenerative changes in the tissues.

CONCEPT MAP EXERCISE

Consult Figure 18.2 (Concept map. Mechanisms of hyperglycemia and hyperketonemia) on p. 476 of the textbook to check your answers.